A Guide to the Spiritual Dimension of Care
for People with Alzheimer's Disease
and Related Dementia

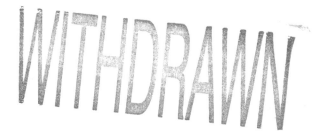

of related interest

Dancing with Dementia
My Story of Living Positively with Dementia
Christine Bryden
ISBN 1 84310 332 X

Alzheimer
A Journey Together
Federica Caracciolo
ISBN 1 84310 408 3

Spiritual Growth and Care in the Fourth Age of Life
Elizabeth MacKinlay
ISBN 1 84310 231 5

Perspectives on Rehabilitation and Dementia
Edited by Mary Marshall
ISBN 1 84310 286 2

The Simplicity of Dementia
A Guide for Family and Carers
Huub Buijssen
ISBN 1 84310 321 4

Reducing Stress-related Behaviours in People with Dementia
Care-based Therapy
Chris Bonner
ISBN 1 84310 349 4

Dementia and Social Inclusion
Marginalised Groups and Marginalised Areas of Dementia Research, Care and Practice
Edited by Anthea Innes, Carole Archibald and Charlie Murphy
ISBN 1 84310 174 2

Ageing, Spirituality and Well-being
Edited by Albert Jewell
1 84310 167 X

A Guide to the Spiritual Dimension of Care for People with Alzheimer's Disease and Related Dementia

More than Body, Brain and Breath

Eileen Shamy

Jessica Kingsley Publishers
London and Philadelphia

First edition published in New Zealand in 1997 under the title *More than Body, Brain and Breath* by ColCom Press, Red Beach.

This edition published in the United Kingdom in 2003
by Jessica Kingsley Publishers
116 Pentonville Road
London N1 9JB, UK
and
400 Market Street, Suite 400
Philadelphia, PA 19106, USA

www.jkp.com

Library of Congress Cataloging in Publication Data
Shamy, Eileen.
   A guide to the spiritual dimension of care for people with Alzheimer's disease and related dementias : more than body, brain, and breath / Eileen Shamy.
      p. cm.
   Includes bibliographical references (p.) and index.
   ISBN 1-84310-129-7 (alk. paper)
   1. Church work with nursing home patients. 2. Alzheimer's disease--Patients-- Religious life. 3. Senile dementia--Patients--Religious life. I. Title.

BV443.5 .S53 2003
259'.4196831–dc21

2002038904

British Library Cataloguing in Publication Data
A CIP catalogue record for this book is available from the British Library

ISBN-13: 978 1 84310 129 1
ISBN-10: 1 84310 129 7

*In memory of my mother, Elsie Elizabeth
Westaway-Fitzgerald, for all people with
Alzheimer's disease and related dementia,
and to honour with gratitude all who care.*

The publishers acknowledge with thanks the kind permission from the copyright holders for the following extracts:

I thank the following for gracious permission to quote copyright material.

Excerpts from *Out of Solitude* by Henri J. M. Nouwen, 1974. Ave Maria Press, Notre Dame IN, 46556. *Head and Heart, Aotearoa*, Psalms by Joy Cowley, Catholic Supplies (NZ) Ltd Publishers. Excerpts from *Caring Alone, Looking After the Elderly Confused at Home*, by Anne Opie, published by Daphne Brasell Associates, 1991. Excerpts from *The Stature of Waiting* by W. H. Vanstone, published by Darton, Longman and Todd Ltd. Excerpt from *The Matriarch* by Witi Inimaera, published by Heinemann. Excerpts from *Hear the Pennies Dropping* and *Tell me the Old, Old Story*, copyright Trustees for Methodist Church Purposes (UK), *The Message, The New Testament in Contemporary English*, paraphrased by Eugene H. Peterson, copyright 1993. Alzheimers disease – *Caring for your Loved One – Caring for Yourself*, by Sharon Fish, Sharon Fish Publications, London.
The Anglican Church in Aotearoa – New Zealand and Polynesia for permission to adapt an anointing prayer and liturgy for the Blessing of a Home (Studio Unit in a Nursing Home) from *A New Zealand Prayer Book*. Robert W. Guffey, author and copyright owner of *Oh to be so Poor* for permission to quote. Excerpts from *My Journey into Alzheimer's Disease* by Robert Davis, copyright 1989, all rights reserved. Liturgical adaptations from *Echoes of our Journey* by Dorothy McRae McMahon, published by Uniting Education, Australia. Hugo Petzsch for excerpts from his occasional paper: *Does He Know How Frightening He is in His Strangeness? A Study in Attitudes to Dementing People*, published by the University of Edinburgh, Department of Christian Ethics and Practical Theology. Quotations from *Humanity Comes of Age, The New Context of Ministry with the Elderly*, by Susanne S. Paul and James A. Paul, World Council of Churches' Publications. Rev. Keith Smith, Executive Officer, Senior Adult Ministries, Uniting Church of Australia, Synod of South Australia for permission to use excerpts from Rev. Dr Elbert Cole's (USA) address to the 1994 National Conference 'Ministry with Seniors', Uniting Church, Australia. Excerpts from *Growing Older* by Dr Una Kroll, HarperCollins Publishers.

Contents

Acknowledgements

This book was written and made ready for publication with the support of many people. I am grateful to the following in particular.

Rev. Max Hornblow, who refused to let the vision of ministry to people with Alzheimer's disease and related dementia die. As superintendent of the North Canterbury Methodist Synod he gave me and the ministry his blessing and a home under the aegis of the Synod. In the climate of that time his was a courageous and prophetic decision.

The Support Group for my ministry, especially Rev. Edwin Clark for wisdom, Elizabeth Hamilton for creative encouragement and Ross Lawn for unfailing loyalty and practical support.

The Methodist Women's Fellowship and the Association of Presbyterian Women throughout Aotearoa – New Zealand for their faith and understanding of the financial difficulties of a pioneer ministry and a non-stipendiary presbyter.

The members of the Dementia Working Group of the Christian Council on Ageing (UK) who affirmed my vision, facilitated my experience and encouraged me to write.

The following people and trusts assisted with the financial support of the ministry and the book: The Christchurch High Street Trust, the Smethurst Trust administered by the Methodist Women's Fellowship of New Zealand, the Media and Communications Endowment Fund, and the Community of Women and Men in Church and Society of the Methodist Church of Aotearoa – New Zealand. Without the generosity of spirit and the vision of those who endowed these trusts this book might never have been published.

Other help was generously given by the Sisters of the Community of the Sacred Name, Christchurch, New Zealand; St John's Parish, Highfield, Timaru, New Zealand and others of ordinary and modest means whose gifts were made large with their love.

This book would never have reached completion without the generous hospitality of these special people: The Sisters of the Sacred Name, Christchurch, who over many weeks graciously provided a safe and prayerful place in their community for me to write; Jill and Canon John Denny who welcomed me within the quiet of their family home while I planned the book and began the writing; Terence and Sonja FitzGerald who cared for me and encouraged my writing through a discouraging and difficult time; Maisie and Maurie Flanagan, who gathered me into the special hospitality of their home

9

and gently let their garden, the animals, the mountains and God restore my energy and spirit whenever that was needed; my family, especially my sons Michael and Stephen Shamy, who cared for my garden and took my dog as their guest whenever the writing or ministry took me away from home – their unconditional love and support, and belief that this book must be written, have upheld me throughout its preparation.

Judy Leonard, graphic artist and friend, listened and then designed the cover of the first edition as a gift.

Finally I owe sincere thanks to Dave Mullan and Colcom Press who took my handwritten manuscript when funds for publication were uncertain and prepared the work for publication in its first edition.

We would like to add our thanks to ColCom Press and to Michael and Stephen Shamy for their permission to publish this latest revised edition.

We would welcome hearing from any copyright owners who have not been traced so that proper acknowledgment may be included in future editions. We would like to thank Catherine Benland for giving permission to use her words in the subtitle of this book – the words 'More than Body, Brains and Breath', come from *The S-factor: Taha Wairua – the dimension of the human spirit*, her submission to the Royal Commission on Social Policy, New Zealand, 1988.

Foreword to the 2003 edition

This book, which was originally published in New Zealand in 1997, was first made available in the UK the following year. It was imported in small batches by the Christian Council on Ageing and, as word of its unique value spread, copies were quickly bought up. Because demand for the book continued and copies had to be printed to order by the enterprising – but small – original publisher, Jessica Kingley Publishers agreed to produce this new edition.

With the agreement of the original publisher and of Eileen's two sons (the author herself unfortunately died before the project was undertaken) the text has been lightly edited to make it more accessible to readers outside the UK. No attempt has been made to excise all New Zealand references – to have done this would have been to risk losing the author's very personal approach. We have simply, where relevant, edited out (or replaced with equivalents) New Zealand statistics and some references to New Zealand organisations and practices.

One of the most notable features of Eileen Shamy's book is the imagination she brings to an area of human experience that was until quite recently seen as beyond the scope of our insight and understanding. That this is no longer the case is largely due to her pioneering work, and tribute should also be paid to the North Canterbury Methodist Synod which first supported and encouraged her in what at that time – the early 1990s – probably a unique mission to people with dementia and their family carers.

As the author remarks in the Introduction, this book owes its being to the fleeting request of an unknown Methodist minister in Manchester in 1992 when Eileen was in the UK lecturing. We should be grateful to this young man, whoever he was, as we are deeply grateful to Eileen Shamy for having given us an inspiring lead in a field that needed, and is happily progressively responding to, such inspiration.

This new edition has been edited by two members of the executive committee of the Christian Council on Ageing, Mannes Tidmarsh and

Albert Jewell, who feel deeply indebted to Eileen Shamy. Mannes heard Eileen when she lectured in England and has been active in promoting the first edition of the book in the UK; Albert, like Eileen, is a presbyter of the Methodist Church.

Albert Jewell and Mannes Tidmarsh
Christian Council on Ageing
Derby, England
July 2002

Forewords

I feel very privileged to write a foreword to Eileen Shamy's thoughtful and sensitive guide to spiritual care of people with Alzheimer's disease and related disorders. The dementias are no longer the forgotten or neglected disorders that they were a generation ago. There is now a huge research endeavour which is bearing fruit in improved understanding of the epidemiology, biochemistry and genetics of these disorders. This has led to the testing of medications that might improve symptoms and quality of life. At the same time Alzheimer's societies have raised community awareness of the needs of people with dementia and their often heroic caregivers.

Despite these advances, spiritual health and well-being of people with dementia and their caregivers have received little attention. In this book Eileen has challenged us all to recognise and respond to this important component without which care cannot be considered to be truly holistic. This book challenges all of us – individuals and health workers need to review our attitudes towards ageing and dementia; the Church must consider the spiritual issues of longer life; and society must recognise and show increased respect for the vulnerable.

This book has a valuable place for all involved in dementia care. Although the author's spirituality is Christian she has 'used words that are acceptable to most world faiths and to those who find the source of nourishment for their spirit outside formal faith/belief structures'. Let us hope that it will lead to a strengthening and enriching of the lives of care givers and those with Alzheimer's disease and related disorders.

Richard Sainsbury, MB, ChB (1972) University of Otago, FRACP (1981)
Professor of Health Care of the Elderly
Christchurch School of Medicine, University of Otago,
New Zealand
October 1997

Eileen Shamy came to the first national conference on meeting spiritual needs of people with dementia, held at York, England, under the auspices of the Christian Council on Ageing. She was a smash hit. Her keynote address was filled with compassion, humour and rugged practicality.

That was in 1991. How did a jobbing psychogeriatrician in a large urban teaching hospital in the north of England become involved in this, perhaps one of the most challenging areas of ministry? Unknowingly and reluctantly would be the brief answer. Here is how it happened. In the early 1990s, I received a letter from Andrew Ferguson, Secretary of the Christian Medical Fellowship. It highlighted the need for an ethical framework for addressing dementia, largely in the light of concerns that the growing debate over euthanasia might encompass people with dementia – the 'slippery slope'.

What was needed, wrote Andrew, was a working party. But who would convene it? Who would chair it? Certain names had come to his mind, and of course one of them was mine. I took the plunge knowing nothing whatever about spirituality in dementia other than what I had recognised in the excellent chaplaincy work in our hospital and the rather striking observation that in our large local church elderly confused people were conspicuous only by their absence.

I set about organising the first meeting of what became the Dementia Working Group of the Christian Council on Ageing. What was extraordinary was that everyone whom I asked to come to the first meeting showed up. It struck me later that right ideas are timely and the spiritual care of people with dementia was one idea whose time had come. Andrew Ferguson was right.

As concerns and experiences were exchanged in the group it became clear that we should organise a conference to bring together those with similar concerns and – more importantly – ideas. Eileen was known to have developed a ministry to people with dementia and their caregivers, something which was as far as we knew unique and certainly needed.

The Dementia Working Group continues, now chaired by my friend and colleague Dr Daphne Wallace. It seemed to several of us as, in the main, professionals involved in dementia care that the secular response to this devastating condition had progressed greatly over the past two decades. In some cases the Church has taken its part, contributing to day care and residential care in some localities, for example. What seemed lacking was a spiritual dimension.

But there was a fundamental theological question, too. Do you, can you, ever stop being a person? This is not such an easy question to answer as may appear, for Western Christianity is both very cognitive and very activity based. What if you become less active and lose your faculties which, after all, is the plight of most people with dementia? In the extreme – and I have come across this only once – the Church itself may cease to treat you as a person on the grounds that you cannot 'get' anything from sacramental worship any more so let's not bother. More subtle and much more common is the unwitting sidelining of confused older people by the church. This is not malign but arises partly from ignorance and fear and also from a confusion concerning personhood.

It was Eileen who introduced me to the simple but marvellously clarifying concept of distinguishing personhood and identity. As the reader will discover, the latter is easily stripped away from someone with dementia but the former endures forever. Why? Because it derives not from us but from God. So simple, so profound.

But the Dementia Working Group has not been concerned with theology alone. A major initiative has been to stimulate the creation of a full-time dementia worker post which has been admirably filled by Larraine Moffitt, based in the ecumenical chaplaincy at Newcastle-upon-Tyne (1995–2000). Larraine is a sought-after speaker around the UK and the ideas behind her post were inspired not least by Eileen's work.

Christ valued vulnerable people but he did not patronise them. So it is with Eileen's book. This is not a textbook nor a theological treatise, yet it informs and offers a practical theology. It is a compassionate book borne out of her own questioning in the face of a mother developing dementia.

Yet it is more. It is a book written by a pioneer. Let me explain. No one would doubt that Christians should uphold and encourage all those involved in improving the quality of care given to people with dementia and their loved ones. We should support our local Alzheimer's group, campaign for justice and better resources and not put up with shoddy care. But we need more. We need Churches to offer ministry, to care for the soul. This is surely something which the Church has to offer which is distinctive. I do not mean that spiritual care can only exist within the churches. I have been moved over and over again when witnessing the interactions which go on between nursing staff on the wards where I work, which often go to the core of spirituality whether involving those who are churched or not. But if the

Church fails in its charge to reach out to meet the spiritual needs of all people by failing those with dementia then it cannot be seen as credible.

This is a book that fills that need. That is why Eileen is a pioneer.

Robert Baldwin, DM, FRCP, FRCPsych
Consultant Psychiatrist for the Elderly
Manchester Royal Infirmary
Manchester, England
October 1997

Introduction

The idea for this book was conceived following a seminar I led for chaplains at Withington Hospital, Manchester in 1992. I had travelled to England from my home in Christchurch, New Zealand, in order to share a way of nurturing spiritual well-being for people with Alzheimer's disease and related disorders. I led a number of seminars throughout England and one at Stirling University, Scotland, and presented a paper at a Christian Council on Ageing conference at York. As a harried, hurrying young chaplain, whose name I shall never know, dashed through the door from that Manchester seminar, he beamed his appreciation and tossed me the challenge of preparing a book: 'Please – I need a book about this! Write a book!'

I heard him but hardly allowed myself to even think of the writing until I realised that I was hearing similar requests from others with a concern for holistic care for older people with dementia. It was especially hard for me to ignore the expressed need of those people who have stayed after my seminars to share the brokenness of their personal experience caring for a loved one with dementia.

I knew from my own experience that Alzheimer's societies throughout the world had raised the awareness of society to the needs of people with dementia and their caregivers. But back in 1990 little or nothing was known or being practised in my native New Zealand to provide for the spiritual dimension of care of those for whom there is as yet no cure.

However, on my return to my work in New Zealand I had little time to husband that seed planted in the Northern Hemisphere. It lay unnurtured in the ground of my mind during most of the busy months of the last half of 1992. Gradually it became clear that possibly the most fruitful work I could do for the future of the ministry I have pioneered would be to write down the knowledge base that I have developed out of my own personal and pastoral experience. So, this book is for all those who believe that human beings are more than just body, brain and breath, and who desire to provide an holistic person-to-person mode of care – including the spiritual dimension – for their loved ones or their clients.

Developing a new ministry from nothing is very different from taking up a new charge in a long-established parish. There were no boundaries, and indeed John Wesley's words 'the world is my parish' were very quickly to become in reality my very own. Writing, educating and advocating throughout my country and beyond it, together with a ministry of word, sacrament and pastoral care to people with Alzheimer's disease and related dementia and their families, have kept me fully extended.

It was not until January 1996, in active retirement, that I was able to give substantial periods of time to finishing this book. In many respects I would have preferred to come to it further down the track. There is still so much to learn. However, I am not at the beginning of my working life. I have come to this work for people with dementia at an age when most are retiring. Now is the time to pass on the modest candle of my own learning and experience in the hope that its light will guide for a little way those that follow in this work.

It will be obvious that this book has been not just a hard writing exercise for me. People with dementia have captured my heart. This book is one consequence of that capture. I hope my readers will be able to understand, if not forgive, my idiosyncrasies and explosions of passion. That passion which may seem to belie a proper objectivity is something I cannot apologise for, although it has put me into some hard places. For one thing, it seems to me that a respectful acknowledgement of affectivity as a valuable human attribute has been an urgent and necessary learning for Western society in the last years of the twentieth century. Certainly people are no happier in my own country because of an enormous respect and reliance upon the cold things of reason and logic, as important and necessary as they undoubtedly are.

> Head said: I am logic. I am structure. I am the stake which supports the young plant. Heart said: I am love. I am mystery. I am the creative force of life. Then Head and Heart begin to quarrel... So Head and Heart went to God and asked if they could be separated. God laughed at them and said: Not even God can do that. You two belong to each other. Apart I'm afraid you're nothing. Head, you are the container. Heart, you are the contents. The container without the contents is as hollow as a drum, all noise and no substance. The contents without the container will disperse and be wasted, good for nothing at all. There is no way you two can be separate and lead useful lives. (Cowley 1989)

As the work I do is but a beginning and as I am not an academic theologian but a very ordinary woman wishing to make sense in the light of faith of all that life, in joy and pain, brings to myself and others I welcome suggestions and criticisms that might be helpful in nurturing spiritual well-being for people with dementia.

During my time in Great Britain and as I go about my work here in Christchurch and other parts of my lovely country I am encouraged by the thoughtful, brave work being done by others to enhance the total well-being of those with dementia. I hope that this book will serve that work and help to bring those who are involved, heart, mind and hands, into some kind of fellowship. Dare I name it a fellowship of the foolish? For foolish we most certainly will appear in a society obsessed by the quantifiable, by the immediate, by productivity and usefulness, by competition and profit, by individualism and loss of community, and where the bottom line really is the bottom line. In that world it is accounted madness to expend precious resources on those who in economic terms are useless.

There is, however, another larger world view represented by a foolish, passionately extravagant woman pouring her alabaster jar of costly, perfumed oil over the head and feet of a man named Jesus – *Tama a te Atua* – Son of God. This kind of costly, extravagant care bears within it a power to heal our own human woundedness. In our hearts we know it, but we need each other's courage and a certain authentic and holy innocence for such foolishness.

Although my own spirituality is Christian, and that will be evident to the reader from the examples I use and the stories I tell, I have tried to use words which are acceptable to most of the world faiths and to those who find the source of nourishment for their spirit outside formal faith/belief structures.

It is obvious that I am not a medical person. My description of Alzheimer's disease is not intended to be a scientific and full explanation, but merely a useful map so that we may walk in some kind of meaningful relationship with people who can no longer remember. Sometimes it will be a scary walk, as we encounter in people with dementia our own monstrous fears of loss and dependence. But there is also blessing. Amid the cruel diminishment of Alzheimer's disease and other dementias I have met the Christ broken and oppressed, and I have loved Him there.

Eileen Shamy
September 1997

1

Through a Door of Hope
or Eyeballing the Challenges

(God says) 'I will…make the Valley of Achor a door of hope' (Hosea 2:15)

How it all began

During the autumn of 1988 my mother died. We had journeyed almost twelve years through the frightening and wearying stages of Alzheimer's disease. While we travelled that journey together, I became more and more distant for my mother. Some days she forgot who I was and some days she confused me with her younger sister.

That is the nature of Alzheimer's disease. And yet, at the end, only three days before her death, out of the dull grey of memory loss and confusion she said to me, firmly and clear eyed, 'God never forgets us. Remember that, dear!'

At that moment her suffering confusion and my weary questioning were shot through with light. The whole devastating experience began to acquire meaning. I knew then that nothing had been lost and that in the end all would be harvest. I am now committed, and others with me, to an unmapped journey, sustained by grace and deep-gut prayer. It is a journey towards holistic care for people with Alzheimer's disease and related dementias in which the spiritual dimension of care is given as much respectful attention as the physical, emotional and social dimensions.

For most of her adult life my mother was a believing Christian, fully involved in the life of her faith community. Her faith enabled her to make sense of life. It had brought her whole through pain and grief and all the significant life-changing circumstances common to human beings. It gave her spiritual health and well-being. In her own way she actively nurtured that well-being in the fellowship and worship of her little congregation until, following my father's death in 1984, we could no longer support her in her own home. The disease had progressed to the stage where she needed 24-hour care. I was unable to sustain that, so with sorrow and irrational guilt my brother and I, with the assistance of a caring social worker, arranged for Mother's assessment and admission to a private nursing home.

There she received care-full skilled attention. There her personhood was respected but there also her fragile hold on remaining observable resources for her consolation and spiritual well-being was broken, lost, forgotten. Although during my visits I would pray the Lord's Prayer and read a little from the psalms or Jesus' words from the gospels, there was in her new home no routine of morning and evening prayer, no grace before meals, no worship or hymn singing which would have helped to keep her faith memory alive.

I share my mother's story, but it is by no means only her story. Increasingly I have found the same 'dying' wherever people are cut off, for whatever reason, from the resources they have used to sustain their spiritual health. When memory and orientation to time and space began to ebb away in the relentless pull of the outgoing tide of Alzheimer's disease, my mother lost the habit of daily prayer and worship. While she was still in her own home she had tried hard to keep in touch with this dimension of her being, walking to her church almost every day because she thought each day was Sunday. But now, 'foxed' by a strange environment and increasing confusion, she could no longer take any initiative at all to attend to her spiritual needs in exactly the same way as she could no longer be responsible for attending to her physical needs.

While much time, money and effort and a large measure of social compassion secure adequate physical care for people with a dementia illness, very little is done to nourish the spirit. Yet the most frequent question I am asked by those who have recently received the diagnosis of Alzheimer's disease and who understand the prognosis of increasing memory loss and confusion is this: 'What will happen to my faith when I can no longer remember?'

It is a very old question. We hear it in the poetry of ancient Israel. 'Are your wonders known in the darkness, or your saving help in the land of forgetfulness?' (Psalm 88:12). God's answer to that desperate questioning was to come among us in the person of Jesus. So genuine was God's identification with our humanity that St Paul could confidently write to the church in Rome:

> I am convinced that neither death, nor life, nor angels, nor rulers, nor things present, nor things to come, nor powers, nor height, nor depth, nor anything else in all creation, will be able to separate us from the love of God in Christ Jesus our Lord. (Romans 8: 38)

If the Church affirms St Paul's claim, it must surely give serious thought and commitment to helping those who are wrapped around in the woolly grey blankets of chaos and confusion to sense that victory.

As I go about my work I find only a small percentage of parish clergy who have considered this, or are confident of filling the need. Fewer still are finding satisfactory ways to minister to seriously memory-impaired and confused people. Most are immobilised by a grave lack of knowledge and understanding of how to provide for and assist their congregations to respond positively to the need for a ministry to people with a diminishing ability to think, to reason and to remember. It is unlikely that at any time there would be more than a few people (and their families) affected by the disease in any one parish. It is only too easy to forget the needs of one or two people. Jesus told a parable about that one lost sheep. My little mother reminds us that 'God never forgets us'.

When I began my ministry to people with Alzheimer's disease and related dementia it was the first of its kind in New Zealand. Subsequently many, both here and in the UK, thought it was the first of its kind in the world. I do not know if that is true or not. What I do know is that nothing existed to help me – no model, no resources, and very little finance. Although there was much goodwill and enthusiasm there was also indifference, prejudice and misunderstanding. The enthusiasm came mostly from the women of the Church who presented me with a substantial monetary gift to help start the work since they understood my call was to non-stipendiary work. Their confidence in the work was a valuable encouragement. In later years, when a prejudiced few in positions of authority lacked vision for the work and actually harmed the ministry, these good friends gave the work the support it needed. But at the beginning – well, where to begin?

Religious ritual

I need not have worried! On the Monday morning, following my Sunday evening induction into this new ministry, 'The Church's Ministry to Elderly and Confused People', I received a telephone call from the motivation therapist working in a large hospital caring for older people. This is what she said: 'Would you be willing to bring the sacrament of holy communion, in the context of a gathered community of people with a dementia illness, most of them in an advanced stage? We have been trying for many years to find a clergy-person who would do this.' Sadly I was to encounter this plea over and over again. Many Christian people with dementia are denied the sacrament. This is a denial of basic justice.

In my tradition, when these old, now dependent, people were baptised the congregation, representing the Church, made a solemn promise to provide for their spiritual well-being and faith nurture. While that promise is commonly regarded as applying particularly throughout childhood and adolescence (that is, the years of relative dependency) it surely does not end there. When these members of the faith family can no longer remember who they are in relationship to God and, indeed, when God's love for them through all the years of their living is forgotten, the faith family, the Church, must remember for them. Through love and practical compassion it should remind them time and time again of God's unconditional love. Henri Nouwen (1998) writes of Christian ministry as 'remembrance' and of the minister as a living reminder of Jesus Christ.

Symbolic action and ritual is a basic normal way of remembering. In both the Hebrew and Christian testaments, remembering (*anamnesis*, that is, remembering to bring the past into the present) is a strong theme. At the beginning of Exodus 13 we are told how ritual can help us to remember. Moses said to the people, 'Remember this day on which you came out of Egypt' (Exodus 13:3) and then he proceeded to tell the people how to do that: in symbol and ritual the Passover observance has served to remind the Jewish people until this day of how the Lord their God brought them out of the land of Egypt and the bondage they had known there.

We find similar ritual in the book of Deuteronomy (Deuteronomy 26:2). This is a harvest festival ritual, when 'the first of all the fruit of the ground, which you harvest from the land that the Lord your God is giving you' is taken to a holy place and given to the priest who sets it before an altar of the Lord. Then the farmer must recite his history: 'A wandering Aramean was my ancestor… So now I bring the first fruit of the ground that you, O Lord, have given me' (Deuteronomy 26:5–10).

Ritual provides an opportunity for us to express our deepest emotional levels of memories and is therefore very important at times of joy, sorrow and celebration, loss and death. In our own time those people who experienced the First or Second World War are deeply moved when the last post is sounded at the Remembrance Day parade. Our rituals are precious reminders which serve to help us towards a renewed awareness of who we are. They establish deep authentic connections in terms of identity as an individual and as members of families, faith communities and cultural groups. Through these rituals and symbols human beings can capture a sense of former self.

Christians are asked by Jesus to re-enact an ancient ritual so that they might remember or bring to mind a memory of him, his life, death and resurrection. The holy communion, the eucharist, as a memorial meal reminds us that memory is a sacrament of hope. Whenever I celebrate this memorial meal with people with Alzheimer's disease or a related dementia I am profoundly moved by their response. So deeply is this sacramental ritual embedded in the faithful Christian's memory, and so powerful is the eucharist as a memory cue, that people who on other occasions show no response whatsoever are stirred and gently brought to the present moment. Hands reach out to receive the bread and on the tongues of many I hear the ancient prayer: 'I am not worthy Lord ... but only say the word and I shall be healed'. The presbyter's task is to be a bearer of remembrance, to re-mind, and so re-member, each person into that place where he or she truly belongs: into the community of God's people.

There are effective ways which can be used to re-member, into their own community, those with Alzheimer's disease who do not profess to be religious but none the less recognise the creator or source of being and, for the sake of their spiritual health and quality of life, can be reconnected to their source of meaning. This book is not only for Christians and other religious people. Although only a minority of the population may claim to be Christian, and far fewer to be practising Christians, most would not deny that they are spiritual as well as physical, emotional and social beings.

Dragons of many names obstruct the way into the Valley of Achor referred to in Hosea 2:15 (the Hebrew word means 'trouble') delaying the promise of hope. It would be foolish not to acknowledge their power over us as we begin our journey into a different kind of ministry. But it would be even more foolish to disregard the power of that compassion which reflects in action the compassion of Jesus. However, there are many negative attitudes which may make it very difficult for people within and without the Churches to engage in a ministry of spiritual well-being to those with Alzheimer's disease and other dementias.

Alzheimer's disease receives a poor press. Much is made of hopelessness, the long drawn out years of dying which many have called the funeral that never ends, the loss of identity, the devastating effects of the loss of memory, the suffering of families and the heavy burden of care givers. Until very recently it would be fair to claim that, on the whole, what the general public heard about Alzheimer's disease and other dementias was the very difficult plight of the care giver. It was concluded that little could be done to improve the quality of life for the person with the disease except to keep him or her warm, clean and nourished.

To focus on the person with the dementia, which is what I believe I am called to in my ministry, with the conviction that quality of life could be vastly improved, raised a great deal of feeling – much of it sympathetic and enthusiastic but some quite cynical and actively discouraging. Even today, eight years later, in spite of increased commitment to holistic care in many rest homes, prejudice, negativity and some apathy remains. If the Valley of Achor is to become the promised door of hope for those in the 'land of forgetfulness', the prejudices and negative attitudes as well as those which are positive must be named and faced with purposeful honesty.

Hearing the music

There is an intriguing story in one of Chaim Potok's novels which may help our understanding of what makes it so difficult for anyone who has a vision of another way of caring to effect change. This story comes from Davita's Harp (Potok 1990). One of the characters, Jakob, tells the young girl, Davita, a strange story about a little bird which woke up one morning in a beautiful land filled with people who were sometimes kind but often cruel. A soft, haunting music could be heard everywhere. It seemed to come from the earth itself, a low enthralling tinkle of sound. The little bird loved the land and did not like the people. He wondered why people made war, why they were so cruel. He thought it might be a good idea to change them. Now how could a little bird do that? One day, as he sat on the branch of a tree in the cool green shade of overhanging leaves, he had an idea. It occurred to him that in some way it might be the music that was the cause of the cruelties he saw. People hurt each other, and instead of feeling sorrow and regret went ahead and were soothed by the music. Perhaps if the music came to a stop; perhaps if there were no music to soothe a person who did harm – perhaps then the harm itself might come to be felt as intolerable and be brought to an end. And so the bird set out to discover the source of the music.

Jesus always put his finger on the source of the music, the tune to which those he encountered danced in spite of themselves. For the rich young ruler it was the melody of the love of money and the good life. But the encounter of Levi the tax collector with Jesus stopped the almost irresistible melody of money. We all have our own compulsive distractions. We all dance to our own music whether it be to the tune of the love of money, busy-ness, prejudice, fear or countless other 'tunes'.

Facing our own music

> Grow old along with me.
> The best is yet to be,
> The last of life, for which the first was made.
> Our times are in his hand
> Who saith 'A whole I planned,
> Youth shows but half; trust God: See all, nor be afraid.'

So writes Robert Browning in his poem 'Rabbi ben Ezra' (Quiller-Couch 1912). But many are afraid. Fear of our own old age may be the dirge that keeps our minds from even thinking about people with a dementia illness. It takes courage to grow old with some sense of celebration, even dignity. 'Old' is definitely not the image most people wish to project and many do a great deal to hide the years.

We can hardly blame them. The last fifty years have witnessed the growth of a youth culture with its own clothes, language, hair-styles and 'in-group' codes of behaviour and acceptance. Gone it seems are many of the intergenerational opportunities of former days. We have seen also the extraordinary phenomenon of the rise of the ghetto-like retirement units and villages. It is now possible to grow up without opportunities for learning to relate to very old people. The effects of this are long term, long term indeed.

The psychological equivalent to the Benmore Dam – a giant hydro-electric dam in New Zealand's South Island – is repression. Repression is a powerful but unconscious force we use to block awareness of certain unwelcome thoughts and feelings. Human beings tend to repress those thoughts and mental images that make them uneasy and anxious. If our inner images of being old cause us anxiety, we simply work hard at repressing all awareness of our own ageing. If visiting a nursing home for aged people makes us feel uncomfortable about old age, our mental processes accommodate themselves to allow us to forget that we have not called to see any of our parishioners or friends and relatives living in nursing homes for several weeks, even months.

The way we think about ourselves and our own old age has significance, not only for our personal lives but also for our spiritual journey and ministry. If we can become aware of and make sense of our own ageing as an inevitable fact extending into the future, we will have more empathy with those persons whose spiritual, physical and emotional needs may remind us of the circumstances of older age. Once we begin to feel comfortable with our own ageing, chronological age tends not to be a factor in our relationships with people. Freed to be ourselves, we relate on the basis of our common humanity.

Recognising and overcoming the fear of our own old age and dependence is an imperative for effective ministry to people with Alzheimer's disease who are usually not only old but also confused and severely memory-impaired. How can we begin to feel comfortable with our own old age? A place to start could be to write down all our negative images and opinions about old people, then try to think of people we know who are old and fit our negative images. Most of us are hard put to find actual people to fit our negative images of older people. Moreover, most people who are difficult at eighty more than likely were difficult people at forty, although perhaps in older age controls and inhibitions are not so strong. If we can identify and deal with our psychological blocks and come to terms with our own ageing we will begin to discover that the chasm separating 'them' from 'us' is not nearly as alarming and wide as imagined. This is not to deny that growing old with dignity and a sense of humour demands courage and wisdom.

Death is another matter. Our own mortality is something we take into ourselves slowly, although awareness of mortality starts very early in life. In my seminars I have often quoted from Chaim Potok's novel *My Name is Asher Lev* (1972). Many people have told me how gently but persistently this incident, remembered from childhood by the chief character, Asher, an artist, has enriched their personal understanding of the two seemingly opposing facts of life and death. Encountering a bird lying in the gutter, six-year-old Asher asked his father if it was dead and, on being informed that it was, he asked why it had died. His father told him that every living thing must die – including Asher's mother and father and in due course Asher himself – because that is how God has made the world. When again asked why, Asher's father replied that it was so that life would be precious, for something that is yours forever cannot be precious.

Life is indeed precious, God's good gift. Gratitude for the gift shows reverence to God in the way we respect not only our own lives but the lives of others.

This introspective discovery of our own mortality gains a social dimension when it is translated into a respect for the precious nature of all human life, young or old, active or passive, useful or seemingly (but only seemingly) useless. This respect is what motivates us to provide for the very best quality of life for all who are unable to help themselves. Unfortunately, some clergy accord little importance to pointing old people towards a Christian understanding and a spirituality of ageing, of loss, dying and death which is positive and motivating. This attitude reflects, even if uncon-sciously, negative thinking about ministry to old people, especially those who are dementing.

I am not alone in my concern. 'Ministry to Senior Citizens' was the theme of a consultation held at the Interface Academy in Pakenham, England in October 1991. This consultation was convened by the World Council of Churches' subunit on Renewal and Congregational Life. It was very clear that the demographic 'ageing explosion' demanded of the Church far more than what was being done through its ongoing programmes. The consultation highlighted the crucial need for congregational education on attitudes towards and care of older citizens.

In a section headed 'The Church and the Elderly' one of the recommen-dations is:

> In all their work, churches must shake off age discrimination – looking upon older people as frail and sick and as objects of care and charity. More old-age homes and hospitals for the chronically sick will not meet the needs of the new era. Instead we must make every effort to include the elderly as full participants, putting an end to ghettoised, old people's programmes. The Churches must join coalitions with other religious and secular groups to press for the broad rights of old people – at the United Nations, international financial institutions and aid agencies and in national parliaments...
>
> Churches must join in the movement to affirm life throughout its lengthening course, keep older persons in the social mainstream – strengthen local networks of caring, building bridges among the generations. Churches must reconsider the spiritual issues and priorities of the new conditions of longer life. (Paul and Paul 1994)

Why are so few doing this? Is it because in our hearts we believe that young people are of greater value than older ones? And if the Church's response to old people in general is so negative, what chance do old dementing people have? Is it that 'music' again which lulls us into apathy, insensitivity and prejudice?

The Music of technology and pharmacology

As early as 1976 Ivan Illich warned that the 'medicalisation' of health care in the United States of America with the consequent neglect of the spiritual dimension was causing enormous increases in costs with no accompanying gain in society's health. There have never been many advocates for the spiritual dimension of being human in my own country. However, in her brilliant submission to the Royal Commission on Social Policy, Catherine Benland (1988) claims that to reject the spiritual dimension, which she names simply as the 'S' factor (*Taha Wairua*), is 'to shatter what should be whole and to obscure what should be clear'. She goes on to say that the social scientists of what many would regard as our secular society have endeavoured to ignore the spiritual dimension, or to explain it away with a new definition using pseudo-scientific language pertaining to the head rather than the heart. She sums up:

> And the technocrats, atheists, agnostics, humanists and cynics who believe that total secularism has been achieved, or is achievable are as much locked into an idiosyncratic unproved belief system as are their adversaries. Their attempt to eliminate the 'S' factor; bypass or repress it; or restrict its meaning to piety religiosity, and superstition are reductionist. Beyond the reach of the human brain and the microscope or telescope is the Tao. You can gild the cage of the well-fed nightingale but you cannot make it sing. And you can't stop the common people continuing to experience and believe in the 'S' factor, and behave accordingly.
>
> Social planners and policy-makers who refuse to admit this may well encounter passive resistance, blocking, failures of schemes and projects and even rebellion.

When the drugs and technology fail to cure, the tendency may be to conclude that all that is important has been done. A notable exception, of course, is the hospice movement, where terminally ill people are cared for with the intention of helping people to live until they die. Drug therapy will, of course, be part of this care, but only as a means, along with other therapies, to improve the quality of life left to the dying person. This has generally not been the case for people with Alzheimer's disease, although their dying may be much longer.

Until very recently their institutional care was based upon a custodial mode, with little emphasis upon quality of life care. If drugs were used it was often more to make life easier for the care givers than to give the patient quality of life. It is likely that confusion and memory loss are exacerbated by such impersonal care. I have witnessed over the recent years the practical expression of a different philosophy of care which tends to be holistic, taking cognisance of the whole person. However, this costs more and today the best profit for investment is an important managerial objective.

Getting the best return for the financial investment through a strategy of improved efficiency is laudable. It becomes contemptible when profit is more important than people. Mercifully there are enlightened, intelligently persistent pioneers speaking out. Quietly but effectively they are conducting courses to provide some training for care-givers or demonstrating the difference holistic, person-to-person care makes to the quality of life for people with dementia. It is now over ten years since I offered the first **day-long seminar for care givers and clergy covering topics such as understanding Alzheimer's disease, the spiritual dimension of care,** communication with people with dementia for relationship building, and more.

The Alzheimer's Society continues not only to support and be an advocate for care givers but also, more than any other organisation, by every means to promote quality of life care for those with an irreversible dementia illness. In the UK I witnessed the forward-looking quality of life care promoted, taught and demonstrated by people such as Dr Robert Baldwin, the founding chairman of the Dementia Work Group of the Christian Council on Ageing; Alison Froggatt (Froggatt and Shamy 1994), the late Dr Tom Kitwood and Kathleen Bredin of Bradford University (1992); Janet Bell and Iain McGregor of 'Spring Mount' (1991); Professor Mary Marshall and her team at the Dementia Care Development Centre at Stirling University (Harrison 1993); Methodist Homes for the Aged (now MHA Care Group) staff, working in some special dementia units; Paul Wilson, a presbyter of the Methodist Church in England; and Evan Millner of Jewish Care. These organisations and individual people work very hard, often against strong defensiveness and financial considerations, in order to raise awareness. They take their philosophy of care very seriously. There will be many others unknown to me whose work I would wish to acknowledge.

Who calls the tune?

There is a disturbing and widely held philosophy abroad today. On every side we are battered into measuring our own worth – and therefore the worth of others – by our ability to pay, by our 'deservingness' before the economy, or by our age. Those in the dependency years, the unborn, little children, the unemployed, the disabled and those over 65, are counted as those of least worth. When human worth is measured by youthfulness, wealth, power and influence, and by education (if it enables a person to earn a lot of money) those not fortunate to possess these 'advantages' become marginalised. However, because these advantages can never be fully secured, many people live with a sense of personal worth which is about as constant and comforting as the dollar exchange rate in a banana republic.

The idols of Western society in this new millennium are materialism and consumerism, and they have us by the tail. We have lost, or are fast losing, the values of 'being'. By contrast, all the major world faiths have steadfastly resisted the identification of a person's worth with their personal usefulness or otherwise to society. Jesus reminds his followers that God's care for the wild flowers of the fields or of the birds of the air is unrelated to productivity. God's love for all people is unconditional, neither limited by our unworthiness nor dependent upon our responses. Just to be is of immeasurable worth to God. Christian people call that kind of love 'grace' because it is unmerited and unmeritable. It is upon this value that the sacredness of all human life rests.

What is very nearly lost when humankind has such mastery of the world (even as I write the ethics of human cloning are being debated) is an understanding of Christian asceticism as practised by those of the Eastern Orthodox tradition, mystics, many conservationists and all those possessing a sense of boundless hospitality. Certainly I am not referring to an asceticism of the hair shirt and other asceticisms of a self-abnegation kind practised by some religious people in the Middle Ages. Rather, I refer to one which is practised in the form of a simple shared life-style, with work done well with joy and generosity and not primarily for personal profit but as a goodwill offering to the whole of creation. It is a kind of natural self-forgetfulness, not an agitation or a self-conscious chore of self-denial or a rejection of the good things of this world created for our use and pleasure. It is honouring and reverencing the creator God and using the good things of this life in simplicity, in sharing and with gratitude. Self-sacrifice and denial are not necessarily life-giving; indeed, it is absurd if we practise an ascetic way of life (even within the meaning I have given it) for the wrong reason or – worse still – mindlessly for no reason at all. Christian self-denial must bear fruit in loving, sharing and concern for others, and I truly believe in a life of contemplative prayer alongside our works of love.

In the present market-driven, user-pays economy the concept of such a life-style is hard for many to grasp. Many will pronounce it as naïve foolishness. It implies something given for nothing, it is in the spirit of costly grace, and it is the good news for our time. However, for many it is too good to be true!

Although in the UK there remains a strong tradition of voluntary work, it does appear to be on the decline. New Zealand society, sometimes including the Church, tends to accord little value or respect to such work. And the danger is that the one who pays the piper calls both tune and dance. During the later years of the twentieth century many social service volunteers in my own Methodist tradition were either replaced by paid professional staff or awarded payment for their work. In many instances the professional social worker supplanted the pastor, and now perhaps we have forgotten the difference! The spiritual dimension of social services and the spiritual needs of both providers and receivers of the services gradually lost importance. Little heed was given to fostering social compassion through volunteer work.

At the same time the parish church began to practise a user-pays policy on the grounds that something like a seminar received without the handing over of money is perceived as of little worth. We were told, 'People appreciate what they have to pay for'. No doubt there is some truth in that, but I am glad Jesus did not instruct the disciples to pay the lad who provided the loaves and fishes for the hungry crowd gathered to hear him teach. Many have lost the gracious custom – let alone the moral responsibility – of sacrificial giving for the well-being of all.

It was not always so. I have vivid memories of my mother putting aside a portion of all her home-made jams, pickles and preserves for 'the work of the Mission'. From an early age I helped her pack all that produce into boxes, and in my child's mind I named those boxes 'God's Jam', 'God's Bottled Plums', and 'God's Pickles', and since we had many gooseberry bushes in our garden I marvelled at God's preference for gooseberry jam. Although my father was often out of work during the depression years of the 1930s it was normal and natural to give away part of all our home-grown and home-made produce to those who had even less. It seemed to me that everyone did so.

Because talents were also included in what was to be shared and my mother was a creative and excellent dressmaker, there was even a 'God's Aprons' box in our home. As a very small child I concluded that God needed aprons. So perhaps it is not at all surprising that I have absolutely no difficulty naming God both Mother and Father.

Of course most of the world's work must be paid for and justly rewarded. I am not saying that somehow our paid work is inferior to our voluntary work – not at all. However, the giving of oneself without expectation of monetary reward is intensely rewarding. Although our human motivation is seldom completely pure and without taint of self-interest, there is a sense in which sacrificial giving involves people meaningfully in the lives of others. In giving we learn about receiving. A healthy interdependence is learned. There is mutuality in relationships which makes it very difficult to ignore the needs of people with a diminishing quality of life.

Jean Vanier, the founder of the L'Arche communities, teaches and demonstrates that it is mutuality of need and weakness which builds community. Independence is such an admired and promoted attribute in our materialistic society that even Christian folk forget that interdependence is the calling of the people of God. Mutuality, our dependence on each other and the whole of creation, makes for a wholesome society and world community where life is more likely to be abundantly good for all.

Dancing the ageism music

Ageism is discrimination against people on the basis of age, irrespective of individual talents and capacities. It is the stereotyping of older people. It is cruel, prevalent and pervasive. Ironically, it is practised by those who, unless they die young, will one day be old themselves and so become the victims of their own destructive prejudices.

All women have experienced discrimination and stereotyping because they were born female. Older women experience a double discrimination because of ageism and sexism together. Since women live longer than men they are generally represented in greater numbers among those with Alzheimer's disease. To be old, female and dementing is very often to be represented as a person completely without worth, a 'nothing' except, as I have sometimes heard it cruelly and crudely expressed, 'a paying bum in a bed'. The bed, of course, is probably owned by a company whose primary aim is to increase the shareholders' dividend. To be old, female and dementing will put you at the bottom of the pile, the last in line when finance, time and expertise are being distributed.

In the Church such people are almost always consigned to the care of other women, seemingly because men have more important work. Among health professionals the care of old and confused people will bring you nothing near the status of those who work in the heart surgery unit or as a nurse in the cancer wards. Not long ago a registered nurse in her early fifties told me that when she was training in the 1960s a harmlessly nonconforming nurse would be sent to work on the geriatric ward as a form of punishment. Consider this true story, reported in the *World Federation of Occupational Therapists Bulletin*, Food for Thought – on Caring (1985). Giving a lecture to a class of graduate nurses the following case presentation was given:

> The Patient: White female. She neither speaks nor comprehends the spoken word. Sometimes she babbles incoherently for hours on end. She is disorientated about person, place and time. I have worked with her for six months but she still does not recognise me. She shows a complete disregard for physical appearance and makes no effort to assist in her own care. She must be fed, bathed and clothed by others. She is toothless so her food must be puréed. Her sleep pattern is erratic. Often she awakens in the middle of the night... Most of the time she is friendly and quite happy. Several times a day, however, she becomes quite agitated without apparent cause and screams loudly, until someone comes to comfort her.

After this presentation, the nurses were asked how they would feel about taking care of such a patient. Words such as 'frustrated', 'depressed', 'annoyed' were used. The lecturer said he enjoyed the care of her and was greeted with disbelief. A picture of the patient was then passed around...it was of his six-month-old daughter.

The question was raised as to why it was so much more difficult to care for the 80-year-old person with identical needs. It was agreed that our perspective must change. Patients ending their lives in the helplessness of old age deserve the same care and attention as those beginning their lives in the helplessness of infancy.

Unfortunately the same negative attitudes exist not only in the health sector and even society generally but also in the Church. In his study of attitudes to dementing people Hugo Petzsch makes a similar point, as quoted in the Church of England Board of Social Responsibility report, *Ageing* (1990):

While it is recognised that many churches would find it practically impossible to accommodate people with dementia in their services of worship it is worth pondering the reasons. A sobering contrast can be drawn between the church's response to people with dementia and to young children. While both groups have in common the tendency at worst to be incontinent, smelly, noisy, and difficult to control, a considerable amount of energy is expended on providing special services for the young and integrating those to some degree into the congregation's main diet of worship on Sundays. It is not difficult to imagine the initial response of most congregations to a dementing adult or elderly person who was brought to a normal Sunday service. The implication of this parallel might lead one to think that the churches are implicitly endorsing a materialist view of humanity. That is, that people are of worth when they hold the ability or potential to contribute to society. While this is the case with children, who are seen as the hope for the future, it is patently not the case with severely demented old people who are not regarded as being incapable of contributing to society.

That there are people within our churches with imagination and enough compassion and ability to challenge this attitude is without doubt. What is needed is an informed leadership and the courage to espouse an unpopular cause, sweeping away long-held prejudices about dependency and older age with a passion that burns for justice, loving kindness and a humble walking with our God who is ever found journeying with the least and lowly. Sadly, the reality is that the patriarchal Church accords justice for women and old people a much lower priority than theological and justice issues such as the ordination of homosexual people, low-cost housing for the poor, reparation for indigenous peoples and numerous other social issues. There are no degrees of justice, although each issue is bound to raise theological differences.

The music of fear

During Alzheimer's Disease Awareness Week in 1993 I led an ecumenical service of worship for people with Alzheimer's disease and other related disorders, their families, friends and care givers. This service has become an annual event and is well attended. The first year I organised and led this service I asked for the assistance of the members of my ministry support group. Some time after the worship one member of that group confessed that she was very frightened and uncertain about her ability to cope when asked to participate. 'I did not know what to expect. I was afraid,' she said. She had asked for her parish presbyter's support, only to hear that he too was afraid. He did not attend. These two friends are not alone in their fear. English deaconess and retired doctor Una Kroll recalls her first day as a medical student on the psychiatric ward, as quoted in *Ageing* (1990): 'I have a vivid memory', she writes, 'of the fear and disgust that overwhelmed me... I wanted to run away.'

Such an encounter confronts us with human helplessness and human vulnerability, with people who remind each one of us of how easily memory and self-awareness can be snatched away. Fear is overcome by compassion and that requires enough imagination to walk in another's shoes. If people with dementia are to be accorded informed, holistic care, those responsible for their spiritual health must take that seriously.

Listening to the music

The demographic ageing trend

Worldwide there are approximately 600 million people aged 60 years and older. In 1950 this figure was only 200 million. By 2021 there will be more people over 60 years of age in New Zealand than children aged 0–15 years. Of all old people in New Zealand, over 90 per cent live in their own homes (Koopman-Boyden 1993). The figures for the UK are very similar.

However, while these statistics are widely available, my own Methodist Church here in New Zealand, in the process of restructuring and planning the future, made little provision for this new context of ministry. Instead, in the minds of some, the criteria for a successful ministry and the successful parish remain as they were in the 1950s and 1960s: a bulging Sunday school and a large, lively youth group. Not only does this ostrich act engender a sense of deep failure and apathy among clergy and laity, it also inhibits an exciting ministry and mission with and for the people God gives us now.

Worst of all, such unrealistic expectations send cruel messages to old people. The future of the Church does not rest with young people. The future of the Church remains as it always has: in the faithfulness of all God's people, whatever their age, and in the very grace of God. The future's respect for older people depends upon intergenerational relationship opportunities now. In my own district the Church cannot fund a ministry to people with dementia but in general continues to find large sums for a diminishing youth work.

During preparation for this book a survey was made of a representative group of ministry training institutions who all said that only very little attention was given to teaching students ministry and pastoral care with old people, and none at all to the pastoral and worship needs of people with Alzheimer's disease and related disorders.

Listening to a haunting and difficult symphony
ACTIVE AND PASSIVE

In his book *The Stature of Waiting*, W.H. Vanstone (1982) asks this question:

> Why is it that, in the professed and public attitudes of today, the proper function of man is identified exclusively with the exercise of his capacity for action, and that his human dignity is alleged to be preserved only to the extent that he acts, initiates and achieves? (p.61)

Our answer to that question may determine the way we respond to people with failing mental powers; people who are not in control, have little capacity for focused action, cannot initiate, who wait upon the world's convenience and pleasure, and are dependent upon others for the necessities of life. Are they no longer in the image of God and therefore without human dignity? Certainly there is the sense that God cannot wait upon the world; God is always subject (the doer), never object (the receiver).

However, Vanstone suggests a double meaning (1982, pp.20–23) which arises out of the Lord's passion and the disclosure of God made by Jesus. It began in the garden with Jesus allowing himself to be handed over to the authorities. From then on he said nothing decisive, he took no initiative for action. By this 'giving over' Jesus gives meaning and dignity to the person with little possibility of focused activity and self-determination. In Jesus' disclosure of the nature of God in his action of 'giving over' we are perhaps entitled to balance the view of a human being perceived primarily as 'fellow worker with God' with the perception of a person as 'fellow receiver with God'.

In a very much wider sense we could claim that the person with Alzheimer's disease is a 'fellow sufferer with God' – he or she is the one who, like God, is 'handed over to the world' to wait upon the world's response.

For those prepared to grapple with these difficult concepts there is the mercy of discovering meaning and purpose in the seemingly wasted and useless 'waiting' of people with Alzheimer's disease and other dementia. For such a care giver the person with dementia possesses dignity and worth.

Dancing the jazz tunes

BUSY-NESS AND A VIEW OF ORDAINED MINISTRY

Many ordained ministers have told me that they cannot find the time to minister to people with some type of dementia. When priorities of time have to be made they choose those tasks likely to give the most return for invested time and energy. In his book *The Contemplative Pastor* Eugene Peterson (1989) writes of a ministry mode which he calls 'contemplative'. This is a ministry mode which I find particularly helpful to those who carry a burden of concern for the spiritual well-being of their people, including older persons with failing mental powers. It is a mode which fosters an holistic approach but recognises that, although many good and dedicated parish pastors try, it is just not possible for one person to do it all. The pastor then makes decisions, consciously or unconsciously, about what he or she does.

Peterson urges ordained ministers to give themselves primarily to the purpose of their ordination. The Church sets aside some of its people and ordains them in order to extract from them a vow that that is exactly what they will be about, namely word, sacrament and pastoral care. This is the promise to which ordained ministers are committed. Their people may most likely forget this and insist upon the ordained person doing many other things to keep the congregation together and out of debt. Some of the things they insist upon, the ordained person will do – but only insofar as his or her main ministry functions (word, sacrament and pastoral care) permit.

Word, sacrament and pastoral care for every man, woman and child in the parish: that is the presbyteral and priestly calling. There are others to sit on committees, to deliver the church magazine, plan the Sunday school fish and chips evening, the seniors' luncheon and all the other hundred and one tasks involved in keeping the parish together. No task is more important to the calling of the ordained pastor than that which John Wesley would have called 'the cure of souls', the spiritual health of the faith community. If the main focus of the presbyter is that for which he or she was ordained, the spiritual nurture and well-being of elderly confused people in the parish take their place alongside the spiritual nurture of all the others in the faith family. All that is required is courage, commitment, some training in communicating with people who have an ever-diminishing ability to think, reason and remember, and above all an obedience to our Lord's command to those who love him: 'Feed my sheep'. 'Busy-ness', 'involvement' and 'multi-focus' are seductive songs with a talent so cunningly clever that we can almost believe we owe it to them to allow ourselves to become harried, exhausted wisps of nothingness.

Listening to the Gospel songs
A MATTER OF FEEDING SHEEP

> When they had finished breakfast, Jesus said to Simon Peter, 'Simon, son of John, do you love me more than these?' He said to him, 'Yes Lord, you know that I love you.' Jesus said to him, 'Feed my lambs.' A second time he said to him, 'Simon, son of John do you love me?' He said to him, 'Yes Lord, you know that I love you.' Jesus said to him, 'Tend my sheep.' He said to him a third time, 'Simon, son of John do you love me?' Peter felt hurt because he said to him the third time, 'Do you love me?' and he said to him, 'Lord, you know everything, you know that I love you.' Jesus said to him, 'Feed my sheep.' (John 21:15–17)

Reading this conversation we are left in no doubt that the strong corollary of loving the Lord Jesus is caring for his people ('feed my sheep').

Now we can be certain that Peter had a fair knowledge of the kind of 'sheep' he was commanded to feed. They would be familiar sheep, fellow Jews. He knew those sheep and he would know how to 'feed' them. He knew the best ways by which to nourish them with God's good news which Jesus had come to share. Peter would know how to communicate with these people who were like himself in a common race, history, culture, religion and experience. But then God took Peter to Joppa (Acts 10). There Peter met a different kind of 'sheep', unfamiliar sheep, non-Jews, 'sheep' that Peter surely never dreamed of being required to feed. Certainly it was a shock, but Peter knew his essential calling. Empowered by God's spirit he went into the house of Cornelius the Gentile and ministered to those gathered there.

Now I think it is rather like that when we are confronted with people suffering a dementia-type illness. These also are 'sheep' of the household of God, but they are strange and unfamiliar to us. We do not know how to feed such 'sheep' or even if it is proper to try. We live during a phase of human history when the fastest-growing age group in the world is that of the 100 years plus group. This means that we can expect an increasing number of people with some kind of dementia illness. These people have a right to spiritual health and well-being. Their spiritual needs are the same as for everyone else. If people with dementia are to sense the love of God we must find a way to remind them and to include them in the Church in spite of the chaos of confusion and severe memory loss. We know from the work of

Brown and Ellor (1981) that the person with Alzheimer's disease (the most common dementia type) retains the ability to feel and respond to feelings. That seems like a good place to begin.

Accordingly we need to develop an understanding of our human-ness that values and respects affectivity along with rationality. Hugo Petzsch (1984, pp.18–20) suggests that there are biblical models to describe some of our attitudes which can be used as metaphors for society's present relationship with those suffering a dementia-type illness. He reminds his readers of the role of the scapegoat in ancient Israelite culture. The scapegoat's role was to distance the people from their sin. Often this is our society's attitude towards those with Alzheimer's disease. People with dementia are stigmatised, marginalised, pushed to the edges of society, and they alone are expected to bear the responsibility for the disintegration of the relationship between themselves and the rest of us. I think this is a worst-case model, but this stance is sufficiently prevalent to be noted. It is evident in the Church but quite unrecognised for what it is.

I hear of clergy who refuse to wear a clerical collar when visiting elderly confused people even when they know that this simple change in clothing could provide a strong memory cue for confused memory-impaired people. These ministers are not willing to accept even that small responsibility towards building a relationship. They distance themselves and resist anything which may bring the cognitively impaired person closer. This attitude is the fruit of extreme liberalism and individualism. It may have been forgiven in a former age when society was church centred and the 'collar' was seen by some perhaps as a symbol of power rather than servanthood. In a post-Christian time others have the power and we have become again what we were called to be all along – servants. People will warm to that symbol.

I find a model for ministry with people with dementia in Mark's record of Jesus' encounter with the Gerasene demoniac.

> They came to the other side of the sea, to the country of the Gerasenes and when he had stepped out of the boat, immediately a man out of the tombs with an unclean spirit met him. He lived among the tombs and no one could restrain him any more, even with a chain, for he had often been restrained with shackles and chains, but chains he wrenched apart, and shackles he broke in pieces, and no one had the strength to subdue him. Night and day among the tombs and on the mountains he was always howling and bruising himself with stones. When he saw Jesus from a distance, he ran and bowed down before him and shouted at the top of his voice, 'What have you to do with me, Jesus, Son of the Most High God? I

adjure you by God, do not torment me.' For he said to him, 'Come out of the man, you unclean spirit!' Then Jesus asked him, 'What is your name?' He replied, 'My name is Legion; for we are many.' He begged him earnestly not to send them out of the country. Now there on the hillside a great herd of swine was feeding and the unclean spirits begged him, 'Send us into the swine; let us enter them,' so he gave them permission. And the unclean spirits came out and entered the swine, and the herd, numbering about two thousand, rushed down the steep bank into the sea, and were drowned in the sea. The swineherds ran off and told it in the city and in the country. Then people came to see what it was that had happened. They came to Jesus and saw the demoniac sitting there clothed and in his right mind, the very man who had the legion; and they were afraid. Those who had seen what had happened to the demoniac and to the swine reported it. Then they began to beg Jesus to leave their neighbourhood. As he was getting into the boat, the man who had been possessed by demons begged him that he might be with him. But Jesus refused, and said to him, 'Go home to your friends and tell them how much the Lord has done for you, and what mercy he has shown you.' (Mark 5:1–20)

Let us now carefully note what Jesus did when this poor, confused, deranged and memory-impaired man (he could not remember his own name), banished from his community to this inhospitable place, came running and shouting towards him. It must have been an alarming encounter, not at all what you might expect on a quiet country stroll. Jesus did not frantically look around for the nearest large rock to hide behind, hoping to become invisible and so avoid this embarrassing man, nor did he send the disciples for a professional (probably a social worker) to take charge of the awkward situation. No. This is what Jesus did: he continued to move towards the distressed man. He asked his name, immediately affirming his personhood. Jesus was not deterred by the man's confused answer but dealt firmly with him as he was and ordered the demons to leave him. Jesus accepted this man unconditionally and that acceptance was the man's healing.

That was not all. When the man was in his right mind (that is, re-minded) he asked to go with Jesus, but Jesus refused and instead reminded him of his friends and so re-member-ed (that is, integrated) him back into his own community. He even told the healed man how to deal with surprised and incredulous family and friends: 'Tell them how much the Lord has done for you and what mercy he has shown you.' And so this man returned to his normal community, not as a person with little self-esteem, suffering disabling chaos, without *mana* or the authority of normality, but as one favoured and blessed by the Lord.

There is something else I want to share about this story. The deranged man's greeting to Jesus is startling. He rushes towards a small quiet group walking in the hills by the sea, and he runs straight to Jesus – not to anyone else in the group – and he addresses this man whom, as far as we know, he has never met before. Furthermore, he addresses him as 'Son of the Most High God'. Is that not remarkable? It seems to support what I have observed many times: people with dementia are not without spiritual awareness.

The stories of Jesus found in the gospels abound with references to such forgotten folk as this unfortunate Gerasene. It seems to have been precisely for people like this that the gospel of Christ was to be such very good news. The Church is the bearer of this good news and yet it seems to be the nature of institutions that they will, if possible, build in protective attitudes and structures to cushion individual members from the discomforts which such embarrassing people engender. But not always.

The song of the community

In the spring of 1992, as the guest of the Dementia Working Group of the Christian Council on Ageing, I presented a paper at a conference in York and followed that with a number of lectures and seminars in towns and cities up and down the UK. At Leeds I was invited to visit the Sisters of the Carmelite Monastery at Woodhall. I gladly accepted.

Some might expect that the Carmelite Sisters and the Methodist clergywoman from faraway New Zealand might have been worlds apart. Not so. This visit remains one of the mountain-top experiences of my ministry. The spiritual nourishment and encouragement I received from the remarkable women of this Community helps to sustain me in my ministry with elderly confused people to this day.

One of the sisters had received the diagnosis of Alzheimer's disease. The Community understood very well the prognosis of confusion and severe memory impairment and the eventual loss of identity and almost total dependence upon others. In spite of all this, they had made a decision to care for their sister within the Community with which Sister E was familiar and within which her remote memories would be deeply grounded. They also wished to do all that was possible to sustain their sister's spiritual health and well-being.

Their decision was a voluntary one and, although they did not count it so, it was very costly. Fifteen women had a living to make, as well as to keep the religious rule and mission to which they were vowed. Now the number available for the work which paid their bills was reduced by three: Sister E herself and a night care giver and a day care giver. It would not be easy for them, and they knew it. They knew also that with this offering of love would come blessing: the blessing of enriched community life, because the weak and the vulnerable, the exposed, those who must wait upon their world's response, are those who are capable of releasing the creative spirit within each one of us to make a place of caring and bonding, a place of precious community, a place where they would go on 'singing the Lord's song'.

In the life of the Sisters at Woodhall I perceive a microcosm of the parish community which responds with informed love and care should one of its members be brought to the chaos of dementia. There is a sacrifice and a blessing. Such a parish will discover for itself that Jesus so often calls, 'Come! Come and be together with my poor little ones'. Then, when we have learned that, he insistently whispers, 'Go, go and tell the Good News'. We had thought we were doing well enough, but then we discern God's secret: those in littleness and weakness have healed us. Life within our faith community begins to move outwards. We are living the Good News!

We are called to discipleship in a time of much noise and clamour. If we are to be heard as a voice for people with no voice it will be necessary to lead not only by example but also to state people's needs cogently, emphatically and with gracious assertiveness. We will also need to understand the nature of dementia illness, especially the most common type, Alzheimer's disease. If we are to minister to people with Alzheimer's disease and related dementia, rather than merely provide a social service for them, we will need to understand not only the nature of dementia but also to think about person-centred, integrated caring, and what is meant by spiritual health and well-being and the spiritual dimension of care. I will discuss these subjects in the next two chapters.

The music of the world may do its best to sabotage our conscience, seducing us to the apathy of, at best, leaving the task to others. But I believe God's purposes for his people in the 'land of forgetfulness' are that Christ's Church remembers them, reminding them that God loves them and never forgets them. This is just one part of the Church's new context of ministry with older people.

2

Understanding Alzheimer's Disease and other Primary Dementias

In her book about Alzheimer's disease Sharon Fish (1990) writes: 'Our brains are indeed awesomely and wonderfully made, but sometimes things do go wrong with this complex computer that controls us, things we struggle to understand.'

The Old Testament prophet Ezekiel was told to take a brick and draw upon it the map of Jerusalem before prophesying against that city. It is always necessary to understand the context of ministry and care before we begin. We need to understand as well as we are able the nature of Alzheimer's disease and some of the more common primary dementias before we can venture with integrity into ministry for people who suffer these diseases.

It is not my intention to provide a detailed study of these conditions. I am not qualified to do that, nor do I believe that it is necessary for the purposes of this book. Of course it is true that the more we know the more likely will be our effectiveness. But it is also true that it was enough for Ezekiel to know the general shape and main communication lines – the walls and main streets – of Jerusalem. It is unlikely that his task would have been any easier or more effective if he had been given a history or architectural treatise.

This chapter is written primarily for clergy, family and nursing home care givers, seminary and ministry students, church leaders, lay preachers, lay pastoral visitors and accredited volunteer visitors who work with people with a dementia illness. It begins with a short overview, designed to give the reader some key information in an easily digested form. This is followed by a more detailed description of Alzheimer's disease and some of the common types of primary dementia. I give a more detailed description of Alzheimer's disease because it is the most common of the primary dementias and the one with which I have had the most experience in caring for my mother and in an extended ministry with elderly confused persons.

Understanding dementia

Contrary to general belief, dementia is not the name of any disease. Rather, it is a name given to a set of symptoms indicating a need for investigation by a competent doctor trained in this field of medicine. Major signs of intellectual and social deterioration are not normal consequences of old age and a reason for such changes in an older person should be sought. Dementia is caused by many things, some of them curable. Other dementias arise from conditions which, as yet, are irreversible, and the person suffering from them is confronted with a devastating prospect. These conditions are called primary dementias and are the principal concern of this book.

Briefly and simply, a primary dementia-type illness causes a decline in a person's ability to:

- think

- reason

- remember.

In other words, there is a general loss of intellectual ability, caused by changes in the structure of the brain. Symptoms included are:

- increasing forgetfulness, especially of recent events

- confusion

- changes in behaviour and personality

- a progressive loss of everyday life skills.

All these will be experienced without the blurring of consciousness, drowsiness or sleepiness that can occur with a reversible dementia.

In many ways dementia is an unfortunate term for the use of lay people because for some it may have connotations of madness. People with a dementia illness may sometimes behave strangely and a few may even become aggressive for short periods if their needs are not understood. However, they are not insane. Rather, they are people with failing mental powers. It is helpful to remember that we accept kidney failure, heart failure, pancreas failure, even bladder and bowel failures, without prejudice. We should not find the concept of brain failure harder to accept.

A competent assessment and investigation is vital for all those with clear signs of intellectual and social impairment. A general practitioner can arrange for this and a social worker with concern and understanding of people with dementia illnesses can be of enormous help in guiding people through the assessment process. If there are difficulties the Alzheimer's Society will give free, sound advice and caring, informal support. Families can be helped to see that they do not need to be put off by comments such as 'Well, what do you expect? After all, she's 75 years old!'.

Not all dementia illnesses are incurable. The conditions causing some can be effectively treated and the old person returned to his or her normal self. Examples of such reversible conditions are:

- depression (of which older people are at greater risk)
- endocrine disturbances, for example hypothyroidism
- adverse reaction to a mixture of prescription drugs
- vitamin B12 deficiency
- chronic subdural haematoma – symptoms of a progressive dementia may not appear until many weeks, even months, after a head injury; however, unlike an incurable primary dementia illness, the patient usually experiences severe headaches and drowsiness, and surgical intervention is crucial – without it death is probable
- slow-growing brain tumours, especially meningiomas involving the frontal lobes
- urinary infections, which in old people may cause some of the symptoms of a primary dementia illness
- chronic traumatic encephalopathy – sometimes known as dementia pugilistica because it is a condition caused by repeated head injuries such as a boxer might experience
- syphilis – at the beginning of the twentieth century neurosyphilitic dementia was the cause of 5 per cent of psychiatric hospital admissions but because syphilis can now be successfully treated with penicillin, neurosyphilitic dementia is very rare
- normal pressure hydrocephalus, a condition which can occur at any age but is most commonly diagnosed in a person's sixth or seventh decade.

Understanding Alzheimer's disease

We will now take a quick overview of Alzheimer's disease, which is the most common type of primary dementia illness.

- It is a progressive illness.
- It is caused by changes in the structure of the brain.
- We do not fully understand what brings about these changes.
- Alzheimer's disease can strike anyone.
- There is no pattern but it is most common among people over 65 years of age. It can also occur in people in their forties and fifties (when it is known as early-onset Alzheimer's disease).
- It affects approximately 1 in 20 of people at the age of 65 and 1 in 5 at the age of 80.
- It has a drastic effect on memory, recent memory being lost long before more remote memory.
- The ability to feel remains long after the person has lost the ability to understand.
- Alzheimer's disease is not a normal part of the ageing process.
- It is not at present curable (although some drugs can delay its progressions somewhat).
- It is not preventable.

We will now explore this brief overview in more detail and follow that with an outline of some of the other types of primary dementia.

In the very early days of my ministry with elderly confused and severely memory-impaired people one woman described her experience of caring for her father with Alzheimer's disease as being like 'a funeral that never comes to an end'. Others have named Alzheimer's disease 'the silent epidemic'. Family members may not be able to pinpoint just when the symptoms began to manifest themselves but once the condition is recognised it can be observed to progress slowly, steadily and insidiously towards severe disorganisation and death.

I do not know when my mother's Alzheimer's disease began but the moment of recognition that something was very seriously wrong with her can never be forgotten. Sharing that moment may help others to understand something of the slow, insidious, relentless progress of the disease. My mother was 73 when my 49-year-old husband died suddenly, in mid-sentence, from his first heart attack. Mother and Father lived an hour from my home in Christchurch and my only sibling, my brother, lived in Wellington, an hour's journey by air. It was a long weekend holiday and I knew that my parents' neighbours were away from home. Although I hesitated to break the news to my parents, knowing they would be alone, in the end there was nothing else I could do.

Recalling what followed for my mother I wonder about the significance of such a shock. I cannot actually remember phoning but I do recall my concern for my little mother because her love for my husband was very great. My parents, of course, came to stay with me as quickly as they could.

I remember that the day of the funeral was cold, grey and thick with a relentless drizzle. When we came back to my home, although there were many people about, it was not difficult to persuade my suddenly much older and somewhat smaller little mother to take a rest. As I settled her in the spare bedroom with a hot water bottle she asked for a cup of tea. She seemed not to remember that she had only seconds before finished a cup in the lounge. At the time, however, I did not register the significance of that memory loss.

Everything appeared to be as normal as it could be in the painful circumstances and I went to bring the tea. I gave it to her, sat down on the edge of the bed and, in the anguish of my grief, said something like: 'Oh, Mum, you have lived a long time. You have known a lot of sorrow. You must have something to say to help me now.' She looked at me strangely. Her face was stiff and her expression as cold as stone. She said, 'I never want to speak to you again. You took my front seat at the funeral.'

I knew then that I had lost my little mother as surely as an hour or two earlier I had buried my husband and father of my children. This strange, cold woman on the bed was not my mother. I wept without control and she did not put out her arms to comfort me.

The point of this very personal story is that I should not have been surprised at what she said. For a long time I had been aware that there were small but definite symptoms that should have prepared me for this kind of experience. My father, who, of course, lived with my mother every day, took even longer to say 'Something is wrong. This woman is very often not your mother'. Frail and tired, he seemed to withdraw slowly into himself after this experience. He could not or would not talk about it. We suffered our sorrow alone.

I think it was harder for my brother because he lived in Wellington and could visit less frequently and usually only for short periods, perhaps an hour after a day's business in Christchurch. Not until he took our mother into his own home for what he insisted would be a pleasant little holiday after our father's death was he able to see for himself how things really were for Mother. Even at that stage she was still capable of presenting quite well for short periods.

That there is an element of denial in delayed recognition is probably correct. However, it is also true that for some the progress of the disease seems so slow and the changes in ability and behaviour so subtle that the full impact fails to register even for those closest to the person with Alzheimer's disease. Looking back I can now see that my mother knew something terrible was happening to her and for a long time worked very hard and successfully at covering up. I am sure that my dad helped her in this. It is not often recognised how hard it can be for families when members in such a situation begin their grieving at different times.

When Alzheimer's disease was eventually diagnosed we had very little understanding of what to expect and where to find information and support. Fortunately these are now available to care givers and families through the Alzheimer's Society, which was founded in New Zealand in 1985 (and has long existed in the UK). There are groups and support networks in all main centres and many smaller towns and rural areas throughout the country. These groups are autonomous, community-based voluntary organisations with a membership comprising care givers, relations and friends of people with a primary dementia illness as well as people working in health and welfare services. Each local group organises its own support system with regular care givers' meetings, telephone support and access to information. The extent of resources may vary but all will provide understanding, caring, listening and care giver support.

Previously, the Society's concern for those people diagnosed with the disease was expressed through its services to care givers and in advocacy on behalf of the person disabled by Alzheimer's disease who needs 24-hour skilled care yet is far from bedridden. Throughout the 1990s and beyond we have witnessed an approach to the care of people with dementia which is more positive. There is an increasing awareness that custodial care alone is depersonalising and limiting. We are discovering more about the disease and its management through research in a variety of disciplines, the work of specialist dementia services development centres, the unique Dementia Working Group of the Christian Council of Ageing and the informed commitment of Alzheimer's Disease Societies throughout the world. We are now seeing a growing commitment to a person-to-person mode of care.

Even so, I have found that mention of Alzheimer's disease will bring into the mind's eye of many people a vision of a helpless, gibbering old man or woman, sunk deep into a chair and restrained either by drugs or physical means. It is therefore important we now look at the stages of Alzheimer's disease and the possible abilities and disabilities as well as some common behaviours of those who must live with it.

The vast majority of older people with dementia live in the community. They are at first only too well aware of the frightening changes the disease is bringing to their lives. The implications of this reality for the Church and others concerned with spiritual well-being are only now beginning to register. It is not true that these people's spiritual needs will be fully taken care of in care homes by local clergy or chaplains (who are few and far between).

Alzheimer's disease is generally described as progressing slowly through three observable stages. Professor Riesberg (1983) has named these as the:

1. forgetfulness stage

2. confusional stage

3. dementia stage.

Knowing the changes that take place at each stage can be very helpful to care givers and those responsible for the spiritual dimension of care. The course of changes in intellectual or cognitive abilities, behaviours and emotions varies from person to person. No two people progress through this disease at the same rate or to the same pattern, but while it is not possible to place a person on the continuum with any accuracy, these stages do provide us with a model for understanding people for purposes of discussion and for planning for the optimum quality of life for individuals living with this most devastating illness.

The forgetfulness stage (minimal to mild dementia)

During this first stage there is short-term memory loss, that is, recent events are forgotten. There is a tendency to forget appointments and objects are 'lost' because the person has forgotten where they have been left. Mathematical skills deteriorate, sometimes dramatically. For example Rev. Robert Davis (1989), who was diagnosed at a very early stage, has recorded, with the help of his wife Betty, that very early he discovered that his mathematical skills were greatly reduced.

These cognitive losses may manifest themselves in a person's performance in paying accounts late, or twice, or not at all. There may be problems with bank accounts as the person has difficulty keeping an accurate record of deposits and withdrawals and balancing the cheque book, bank and credit card statements. An anxious attention to the diary or calendar may be observed as the person endeavours to beat failing recent-memory ability and maintain a comfortable measure of self-esteem. Abstract thinking shows some impairment and the person may fear or resent the unexpected. Sometimes a previous zest for living is lost and a general apathy and weariness is experienced. Emotional changes such as anxiety and an uncharacteristic irritability may be felt.

Denial, manifest in suspicion – especially of the one closest to them – may be used as a defence against the emotional trauma of losing one's intellectual abilities. For a while the person may turn against the one closest, with hurtful and untrue accusations of theft of personal belongings and money. Relatives, neighbours and friends, and even the minister or priest, can frequently take these stories of 'the terrible dishonesty' of a son, daughter or spouse seriously. That can of course be very hurtful for the person doing his or her loving best to care and understand. Usually at this point, if it has not already been done, a diagnosis will be sought.

However this is not as easy as it may seem. Quite often, the person at this stage of the disease maintains there is nothing to go to the doctor about, and stubbornly refuses. That is when a wise social worker can help. He or she will know that a person with Alzheimer's disease at this stage is often capable of presenting very well for the usual maximum 15 minutes of the doctor's consultation time. Added to this difficulty is the fact that generally the person will look the picture of good health.

The priest or minister without this knowledge can be downright unhelpful. I have known care givers to whom it has been suggested that they are the ones needing the doctor's attention. Of course, no one ever means to be so unhelpful, even damaging; however, such misunderstandings do point to the responsibility that all those with caring and pastoral responsibilities have to take measures to be adequately informed.

The confusional stage (mild to moderate dementia)

This stage is generally the longest and, according to some sources, may continue from two to ten years. It is characterised by increased memory loss and confusion. Families may be astonished, hurt and dismayed when their relative complains or upbraids them fiercely for never visiting when in fact they may have visited the previous day or even just a few hours previously. Gradually disorientation to time and place becomes more and more disabling so that the person may get lost in his or her own home or garden, not know the name of the day or the morning from late afternoon, and forget the names of people he feels he knows. He may not even remember the faces of close friends. Although the remote memory is eventually lost it is the recent memory that increasingly deteriorates the most.

In this confusional stage the sufferer may experience bouts of extreme restlessness and agitation although she will be unable to explain their cause. A woman may incessantly turn out cupboards and drawers as if searching for something. There will be increasing difficulty in thinking logically. Needed words cannot be recalled so that there may be a tendency to withdraw into silence or fill the blanks inappropriately. Judgement deteriorates so that driving ability is seriously affected. Foolish, even disastrous, decisions may be made. Heightened confusion may cause disruptive behaviour, aggression, unrealistic demands and wandering.

Those skills learned most recently are the ones lost first, so an immigrant, learning a new language in adulthood, may revert to his first language, unable to use the acquired, second language even though he or she may have used it for a long time. Work and hobby skills will be among the first to be eroded and perhaps eventually lost altogether. Although there may be the odd spasmodic flare-up of weeping or irritability, the mood generally is flat. To conceal failures of memory the person may use arguing, defensiveness and confabulation. In this confusional stage he or she may wander at night and want to sleep during the day. All sense of time and routine will eventually go, so that meals are forgotten and personal hygiene neglected.

Gradually the care giver comes to realise that 24 hours of constant care are required. Few care givers can or should be expected to provide that. The sad trauma of transferring care to professional care givers has begun.

The dementia stage (moderate to severe dementia)

This stage is reached when remaining intellectual and self-care abilities have deteriorated to such an extent that they can no longer sustain survival if the person were to be left alone to fend for himself or herself. Many people with Alzheimer's disease may never reach this stage because they die of other conditions (heart attack, stroke or pneumonia, for instance) before the disease has progressed this far. Much depends upon the age of a person when the illness first strikes, as well as upon other factors of general health. My mother, for instance, died from a stroke in her eighty-sixth year. Her Alzheimer's disease had reached the stage where, while she generally recognised me (or if she did not, she was at least consistent in regarding me as her younger sister!), she could not have survived alone because she would not have remembered to eat and drink or to exercise caution with electricity or fire or other matters of day-to-day living.

Those, like Robert Davis (1989), who was in his early fifties at the onset of his illness, tend to suffer a much faster rate of the disease's progression and consequent deterioration. In older people this stage may last from one to three years. In this time there is gross destruction of all intellectual capacities, complete or near-complete loss of insight and recognition of self, as well as physical wasting, with consequent weakness. This renders the person even more dependent as help is needed to walk.

As the disease relentlessly continues to destroy the brain, the immune system is compromised and the patient becomes vulnerable to infections. Pneumonia is often the immediate and merciful cause of death.

While progress through each of these three stages is gradual and remorseless in its destruction, a surprising number of 'islands' of relatively normal activity will be noted by the observant care giver until late in the process. We do not know just which functions may remain intact or for how long. Personal characteristics and history will mean that each person will be different. It is very important that care givers know this and understand that recognition of these 'islands' of abilities and their encouragement is crucial to making the most of them, no matter how small.

However, in my opinion the most significant factor in determining a better quality of life is this: feelings remain intact long after the person has lost the ability to understand. This, and the knowledge that remote memories can be triggered or cued, are powerful positive factors which can assist all those who in compassion choose to walk with the patient through the sad maze called Alzheimer's disease.

Other primary dementia diseases

Multi-infarct dementia (MI-D)

MI-D is caused by a series of mini-strokes and is characterised by its abrupt onset, stepwise deterioration and fluctuating course as improvement occurs after the first cerebral infarct and then deteriorates again following the next one. After Alzheimer's disease MI-D is the most common form of dementia.

The cerebral infarct causes confusion and loss of specific cognitive functions such as aphasia, agnosia or apraxia (see 'Some terms' below) according to the intensity and location of each mini-stroke. These losses may be accompanied by weakness down one side of the body. The person suffering MI-D has less control over his or her emotions and weeping for little or no discernible cause is common, as is depression.

Alcohol-related dementia

Prolonged abuse of alcohol can in some cases lead to a progressive dementia similar to Alzheimer's disease. The main features include decline in general intellectual abilities, memory impairment, emotional instability, loss of skills necessary for self-care, and possibly delusions.

Alcohol-related dementia is not the same as another alcohol-induced condition known as Korsakoff's disease, which is also characterised by memory loss. Korsakoff's disease affects a person's recent memory to the extent that there is no recall of what may have happened only seconds earlier.

Creuzfeldt-Jakob disease (CJD)

CJD occurs in approximately one person in every million people. It is so rare that I include it here only because of the publicity it has received in recent years in connection with so-called 'mad cow disease' in Great Britain. This has brought it to the notice of those who, in all likelihood, would otherwise have remained blessedly ignorant of its existence. Once evident, this dementia progresses very quickly. The first stage of the dementia is characterised by extreme tiredness, an unsteady manner of walking and emotional instability. Eventually the sufferer may develop a severe mental disorder in which his or her contact with reality is grossly distorted.

Pick's disease

This dementia is very difficult to differentiate from Alzheimer's disease until the brain can be examined after death. Pick's disease, however, is characterised by confabulation, very silly emotion and loss of inhibitions. The memory and intellect remain relatively intact, although the more obvious changes in personality often overshadow any loss of intellectual abilities. In this it is different from Alzheimer's disease where changes in cognitive function are noticeable early.

For further information on Alzheimer's disease and other forms of dementia see the reading list given in Appendix 1.

Conclusions and implications

These brief and simple descriptions of irreversible dementia illnesses are no more their sum than a map of the Pennine Way is the sum of the experience of walking the track itself. They provide the reader with no more than a map indicating the context of caring. A map is not the journey. Ezekiel's clay map was not the mission.

A map begs questions and decisions. Do I want to make this journey? What is my purpose or destination? Shall I take this route or will I travel that road? Why? How will I travel? Do I need a guide and companion or will I be travelling alone? What will it cost me? What or who will hold me if the way becomes rough or even dangerous? These are questions that must be faced by each person who contemplates a call to journey with people with Alzheimer's disease or a related dementia illness.

For me, the purpose of the journey is quality of life for each person, the mode is one of holistic or integrated care, and the particular road I am called to travel is that of the spiritual dimension of care. The concept of 'holism' is by no means new. Eighty years ago Alfred Adler (1921, 1924) wrote of taking an holistic view of the needs of clients. While many different authors have conceptualised this philosophy differently, they all discuss the nature of a person as having several different dimensions. These include the physical, the emotional and the social self and what has sometimes been referred to as the 'fourth dimension', that is, the spiritual self.

Adler's important contribution was to highlight the difficulty of trying to address each dimension as if the others did not exist. The concept of holism advocates the inclusion of all four dimensions in any care mode. In terms of care policy this means that care home management must address the spiritual needs of its patients and residents. It is not enough merely to arrange for clergy to provide worship opportunities; there must also be training for staff to develop their capacity to interact with the patients and facilitate articulation and insight into the whole being. We know now that people begin to die when the human spirit lacks nurture and well-being.

Chapter 3 will deal with the spiritual dimension of care for people with Alzheimer's disease and other dementia illnesses, but before we turn to that central theme a list of definitions may be found helpful.

Some terms

Some understanding of the language used in describing particular behavioural difficulties experienced by people with Alzheimer's disease and other primary dementias is necessary for all those working with confused elderly people. Here is an explanation of some of the language of neuropsychology as described by Stokes and Goudie (Holden 1990). Although all parts of the brain have a role to play in conjunction with other parts in producing behaviour, it does appear that there are areas of specific localised function, for example, speech is usually centred in the left hemisphere. However, it is the frontal region which is of special interest to those working with confused elderly people because damage there can cause troublesome behaviour. Of course, not all these disabilities will be present in each patient; they vary from person to person.

- *hemisphere*: the human cerebral cortex is divided into right and left hemispheres

- *dominant hemisphere*: the hemisphere referred to as the dominant hemisphere is the more important one of the two hemispheres for comprehending and producing speech; it is usually the left hemisphere, especially in right-handed people

- *lobe*: each of the two hemispheres is divided into four parts; each area is called a lobe. Each hemisphere has a frontal lobe, a temporal lobe, a parietal lobe and an occipital lobe. The division of each lobe is based partly on anatomical factors and partly on functional aspects

- *cerebral cortex:* the outer sheath of the human brain

- *neuropsychology*: the term used for the study of the relationship between behaviour and the brain

- *acalculia*: the term used specifically for number problems

- *agnosias*: these relate to disorders of recognition, that is, the inability to identify an object by sight alone, and speech or sounds by hearing alone. The following are the most common agnosias:

    (a) *anosognosia* (sometimes called left side neglect): with this condition the person may not 'see' his or her own body as a whole, and may deny that the left arm – or other part – belongs to him or her. It may be regarded as a 'foreigner' in bed with the person

    (b) *prosopagnosia*: an inability to recognise familiar people, for example, a spouse or daughter. Sometimes the person with prosopagnosia is able to resolve this difficulty once the familiar person speaks. The familiar voice is recognised

    (c) *simultangagnosia*: an inability to recognise writing and pictorial material as a whole; only parts can be recognised

    (d) *spatial agnosia*: an inability – not caused by an impairment of the memory – to find one's way around familiar places

    (e) *visual agnosia*: the inability not only to name or use an object without touching it but also to recognise that object's meaning and character. That is to say, a person seeing a comb on the dressing-table not only does not know what to do with a comb but cannot even remember having seen anything like a comb before

- *agraphia*: used to refer specifically to writing disorders

- *alexia*: refers to reading difficulties

- *anomia*: describes difficulty in finding words

- *aphasia*: refers to an impairment of language. Often this term is used simply to describe speech impairment but it really includes reading, writing, comprehension and numbers as well

- *apraxia*: movement disorders, not caused by physical deficits. The person is able to move and can perform actions without thinking but runs into difficulties when a conscious attempt is made to perform a particular task. For instance, in dressing apraxia the almost automatic routine of dressing oneself is lost because of brain damage in the non-dominant parietal and occipital lobes, resulting in the person becoming unable to relate themselves to their clothing; clothes are put on upside-down, back to front or in the wrong order.

Suggestions for further reading will be found in Appendix 1.

3

The Spiritual Dimension of Care

Are your wonders known in the darkness, or your saving help in the land of forgetfulness? (Psalm 88:12)

What paltry nourishment is provided by reason alone. (Source unknown)

Ah, mokupuna, but your life began even before you were born in Waituhi. Ara, you have eternity in you also. (Witi Inimaera 1986)

[God] has made everything suitable for its time; moreover he has put a sense of the past and future into their minds. (Ecclesiastes 3:11)

In 1989 in San Antonio, Texas, I spoke with an Anglican priest of the Navajo Nation, the indigenous people of that part of North America. He told me that the average life expectancy of Navajo males is 40 years. I asked the reason for such early death and was told that the statistics would cite alcohol-related diseases as the main cause and that would be correct. But, in his view, there was an earlier 'dying', the death of a man's spirit.

'Oh, yes,' he said. 'The dole cheque arrives regularly on the reservation. The belly is full, but life is such that the means by which my people have nourished the spirit have been lost, denied and denigrated. For them there is no meaning and purpose in life. They die.'

In his book *Man's Search for Meaning* Viktor Frankl (1963) concluded that those who were able to survive the Holocaust were generally characterised by an inner spiritual strength and will to live. An unknown poet in such circumstances wrote:

The sun has made a veil of gold
So lovely that my body aches.
Above the heavens shriek with blue
Convinced I've smiled by some mistake.
The world's abloom and seems to smile,
I want to fly, but where, how high?

If, in barbed wire, things can bloom
Why couldn't I? I will not die.

Anne Frank (1960) did not survive the Nazi Holocaust but left abundant evidence in her diary that even in the most difficult and dangerous circumstances life was fundamentally good. There was something indefinably more than could be seen or measured. In almost the last entry in her diary she wrote:

> I still believe that people are truly good at heart. I simply cannot build up my hopes on a foundation consisting of confusion, misery, and death. I see the world being turned into a wilderness, I hear the ever-approaching thunder, which will destroy us too, I can feel the suffering of millions and yet, if I look up into the heavens, I think that it will all come right, that this cruelty too will end, and that peace and tranquillity will return again. (p.220)

Such a strong affirmation of life in the face of such devastation does not come from human intellectual reasoning but from the strength and brightness of the human spirit. There is a spiritual dimension to every life:

> We are more than body, brain and breath. There is something more which, although it defies measurement, has such reality and importance that to discount it is perilous and to provide for it is good. (Benland 1988)

In her wise and insightful submission to the Royal Commission on Social Policy in 1988, Catherine Benland names that 'something more' simply as the 'S' factor. It stands for:

> something real – something witnessed to and experienced since pre-history. Maori sum up this 'something' as *taha wairua* (literally the side, or aspect of flow that is deep, insubstantial and spiritual...it has no boundaries). (Benland 1988)

Within Western culture there is a strong tendency to separate body from soul. We have inherited the Greek understanding of being human as being two separate entities: body and soul. In this understanding it is the soul which seeks for God, the Transcendent, the One 'out there'. Body and soul/spirit have been seen at some periods of church history to be in combat with each other. Soul or spirit was definitely of more worth than the body. Such an understanding has sometimes led to cruel moral judgements which came into sharp focus in the days of witch hunts in the name of Christianity. The ancient Hebrews did not view things in this dualistic way.

It must also be recognised that for most people there is a very real confusion between 'religious' and 'spiritual'. Many will acknowledge that they are spiritual beings but deny that they are religious. 'Religious' means relating to or having reference to religion, which is a framework of theistic beliefs and rituals giving expression to spiritual concerns. The word 'spiritual' embraces the essence of what it means to be human. It involves right relatedness and includes those experiences in life which transcend sensory phenomena. It is concerned with personhood, identity and the meaning of life. It is impossible to describe completely or to quantify and measure. The spiritual integrates and holds together the physical, psychological and social dimension of life. It integrates these three dimensions into an individual person who is more than the sum of his or her parts.

Health care which fails to include the spiritual dimension treats people as less than human. The United Nations sponsored World Assembly on Ageing in 1971 affirmed spiritual well-being as a basic human right. Neglect of the spiritual dimension of care seriously impoverishes the quality of life for people with a primary dementia condition just as surely as neglect of the physical dimension, although the latter may be more apparent.

Although I write of the spiritual dimension of care it must be made very clear that spiritual care and well-being cannot be separated from the physical, psychological and social dimensions. It is not enough to plan for freedom of religion and worship separate from the rest of living. We are concerned with the whole person. That which is not whole is broken.

There are many broken people in modern technological society. Some, like Humpty Dumpty, may never be put together again (not in this life, anyway). But the wise and grace-filled nourishment of the human spirit, open to the invitation of the divine Spirit, may be healed to the extent of becoming a rainbow for others. Making rainbows of human lives is surely the mission of the faith community. It has much to do with that 'pain in the neck of his people', the prophet Micah, who thundered out in the interests of the little people in the little places: 'God has told you, O mortal, what is good, and what does the Lord require of you but to do justice and to love kindness and to walk humbly with your God (Micah 6:8)'.

Spiritual well-being

In the course of my ministry with people with serious brain failure through dementia illness I have sought an understanding of spiritual well-being which is inclusive. Organised religion is only one way of nurturing spiritual well-being. The practice of religion does not necessarily guarantee spiritual health and life. Christians at least must confess that the practice of religion as taught in particular times and places has eroded self-esteem and placed unwarranted importance on economic productivity and social roles. Far from encouraging human maturity, inner connectedness and harmony, it has often brought people to old age in fear and guilt.

In 1991 I addressed and led discussion with nearly two hundred different groups. My objective was to raise awareness of the importance of the spiritual dimension of care for people with brain failure such as Alzheimer's disease and other types of irreversible dementia illness. I went to all kinds of men's and women's clubs, such as Lions and Rotary, Probus, bible study and prayer groups, house churches, discussion groups of many kinds, groups of nurses, activities officers and occupational therapists, young people's organisations such as Guides, groups for the middle-aged, hobbyists and disabled people – you name it, if I was invited, I went. I went to people in cities, small towns and rural communities, literally in sunshine, rain, wind and even snow. At all these clubs and groups I asked people to share with me their understanding of spiritual well-being. They knew about physical well-being, especially when it had temporarily departed. Generally they were mostly aware of their own emotional well-being in simple terms of happiness or misery. But were they in touch with their own spiritual dimension of being?

The answers amazed me. Only the very young gave me 'churchy', religious answers, and I suspect that was because they knew I was a clergywoman. I found it tremendously interesting as the year went on to realise that, although most people expressed their ideas differently – some with elegance and others, perhaps unused to such abstract concepts, hesitantly and in very down-to-earth and colloquial language – all were saying the same thing. One person affirmed life with a loud firm 'yes', another 'hurrah for life'. Some people described their concept of God in expressions such as 'life-force', 'creative power', 'source', and two said 'the joker up there'.

Eventually I put together a definition of spiritual well-being true to all those contributions: spiritual well-being is the affirmation of life in a relationship with God, self, community and the environment that nurtures and celebrates wholeness. It is the strong sense that I am 'kept' and 'held' by someone greater than myself who 'keeps' the whole of creation, giving life meaning and purpose. It is the certain knowledge that I am part of that meaning and purpose.

Habakkuk's prayer, born out of an ancient agricultural economy, could be a similar expression of spiritual well-being:

> Though the fig tree does not blossom, and no fruit is on the vines; though the produce of the olive fails and the fields yield no food; though the flock is cut off from the fold and there is no herd in the stalls, yet will I rejoice in the Lord; I will exult in the God of my salvation. (Habakkuk 3:17)

Some, familiar with such theories, may find understanding of the meaning of spiritual well-being from the perspective of closely related concepts. A state of spiritual well-being could be said to closely parallel Erikson's (1963) stage of ego integrity or Maslow's (1954) hierarchy of self-actualization. McClusky develops another hierarchy, the final level of which deals with the need for transcendence or going beyond the self in order to find meaning in life (Grabowski 1981).

My own 'vox-pop' definition of spiritual well-being involves three essential factors: a sense of identity, a sense of relationship and a sense that life has meaning and purpose.

Viktor Frankl (1963) claims that life may be made meaningful in a three-fold way.

1. By realising (that is, fulfilling) creative values, for example, achieving a task like baking a cake, painting the house, planting a garden, drying the dishes, and so on.

2. By realising experiential values, for example, experiencing the love of at least one other human being – perhaps even a pet – and experiencing the good, the true, the beautiful, for example, music, poetry, art and nature. St Paul, of course, knew this long before Frankl. Writing to the Church at Philippi he exhorts the people in these words: 'Finally beloved, whatever is true, whatever is honourable, whatever is just, whatever is pure, whatever is pleasing, whatever is commendable, if there is any excellence and if there is anything worthy of praise, think about these things' Philippians 4:8.

3. By realising attitudinal values, that is, making sense of or accepting without despair and disintegration whatever undeserved suffering life may throw up. This nearly always implies some kind of faith system and is where religious belief and practice enter the picture.

A very good example here would be Habakkuk: in spite of the worst natural calamities that can face an ancient agricultural economy, he continued without despair to praise his God and affirm life. Most people would be able to identify someone they know who has been able to rise above undeserved suffering without despair or bitterness; one who is still able, in spite of the cruellest circumstances, to embrace life positively.

The challenge for care givers and pastors is: how can we nurture this well-being in the person who has a diminishing ability to think, to reason and to remember? Certainly it seems unlikely at this stage of our understanding of Alzheimer's disease that it is possible to advance spiritual growth in such a person – although Christians would want to add that it is never possible to discount the work of God's spirit in anyone's life. What we can do is try to make available that which has always been present and part of a person's spiritual life and well-being.

Conserving skills

I spent many years as an active educationalist, deeply interested and actively involved in the way in which children learn to read. As a teacher of early reading I had seen the developmental blocks of learning being put into place and built up in the child. As each new skill was mastered another block was put in place. Before that could happen, however, it was necessary to recognise and consolidate existing skills.

Working now with old people with failing mental powers I seem to be observing the reverse process. The developmental blocks are slowly being dismantled. Even so, the same principle applies: what abilities remain? Care givers must recognise and provide opportunities for using remaining skills. I call this 'habilitative' strategy – one works with what is there. It is important to recognise remaining skills and abilities rather than lament the deficits.

Of course, eventually the skills presently used by a person with Alzheimer's disease are lost and another developmental block has disintegrated. Once again the question is: what are the remaining skills? What is left? I believe that skills are too often lost before their time because the primary focus in some nursing homes for people with dementia is custodial rather than habilitative; staff are not trained to recognise and nurture individual abilities. This is especially so during weekend care when care giver staff changes. Often this is when part-time workers are brought in and activity programmes are suspended until Monday. Some care homes provide for an activities programme for only part of a week.

As an example of the deprivation this can cause I think of my mother who had always been a talented needlewoman and craftsperson. Her hands were never idle. When she went into a care home because she needed 24-hour care she was still crocheting. She crocheted squares for Afghan quilts and her work, even then, was some of the most perfectly executed that I have seen. She took pleasure in the colours, arranging them harmoniously and crocheting the squares together. That she found the work satisfying was obvious. It seemed to me that the fact that her hands were always busy was the reason she seldom wandered or showed any impatience with being confined to the house or garden.

One weekend when it happened that I was not well enough to visit, she dropped her hook and could not find it. All that day, on and off – I was told afterwards – she picked up her work and asked for her crochet hook. No one thought it important to look for it and the weekend staff did not know that she had a spare hook in her room. She still had her work-basket in the lounge on Monday when I visited again. Immediately I noticed her still hands. I picked up the partly completed quilt and she began to cry. Why was she crying? A passing regular staff person remarked, 'She hasn't crocheted all day. Weekend staff told us that she was very agitated most of Saturday and Sunday. The cook said that she had lost her crochet hook.'

I went to fetch the spare hook from her room and placed it in her hands. She looked bewildered, so I took it and crocheted a few stitches. I told her that she was much, much better at this than I was. But when I placed the hook in her hand she held it awkwardly and poked it aimlessly, not even connecting it to the wool. Silently she put it down and folded her hands. She never picked it up again. It was a kind of dying. I grieved for her loss.

Why had none of the weekday staff thought to fetch her spare hook? If I had been well enough to visit her that weekend would she still have been crocheting? If she had dropped her soup spoon someone most certainly would have replaced that for her. I was right to grieve. She remained sad and restless and her little hands stiffened without the exercise. Worse, another resource for nourishing her spiritual well-being was lost to her. Her last remaining creative skill, her opportunity to make something useful which had helped to give her life meaning and purpose, was gone – and those who were her care givers did not recognise the extent of her loss.

How could they? At that time most non-registered nurse care givers hardly understood the nature of Alzheimer's disease, let alone the spiritual dimension of care. Mostly they were good, kind women, but training for their caring work was not required. Many untrained care givers have a natural intelligence and sensitivity, and gladly and eagerly embrace all the information they can acquire. Only very recently has the need for training been recognised and it still depends on the value care home management places on in-service education. A custodial mode of care is less costly and in a profit-driven economy makes more sense.

The situation regarding training remains unsatisfactory. Care workers receive little formal education for their work and very few care homes will pay the cost of employing trained and qualified occupational therapists. The situation is improving somewhat with the institution of NVQs and should improve further with the implementation of new government care standards. However, it will be a long time before the significance of providing opportunities for people with dementia to regularly practise remaining skills is recognised in all dementia care facilities. Nor must it be forgotten that 70 per cent of all people with a dementia illness are cared for at home and as yet there are no formal training opportunities at all open to 'at home care givers'.

The feel of Alzheimer's disease

Robert Davis is a Presbyterian minister in the United States. In his early fifties he was diagnosed as suffering from Alzheimer's disease. His diagnosis was made at an early stage in the progress of the disease. With the help of his wife, Betty, he records his journey into this devastating disease (Davis 1989). At the time he began his record he could no longer remember a list of more than five items, nor read even simple magazine articles. All his mathematical skills had gone, he became lost and confused in familiar places, and his IQ had dropped to half its former level.

He writes (pp.121–123) that the first spiritual change he noticed was fear – he is unable to reach comforting memories. A man of prayer, he found it difficult to pray at all. His former sense of the companionship of the Holy Spirit has faded. He writes that he feels like an orphan child, alone, lost, deserted, abandoned and never found again. He is often very frightened and tells us that he is comforted at such times by loving reassurance, soft touching and a quiet, gentle voice with soothing words.

Change and the loss of his life-long spiritual resources which sustained him in life's hard places give great grief. No longer can he use his Bible and find there God's revelation for himself and his world. He tells us that he is exhausted reading the same two or three verses over and over in a vain effort to retain the sense of what he has just read. The ability to pray, which in his tradition is intellectual and word-filled, was impossible to claim. The modern sacred music which previously provided spiritual joy no longer does so. He tells us that now his God is revealed to him in the creation (pp.131–132). He is brought closer to God watching nature videos than by the Sunday morning sermon which is a jumble of twisted ideas and meaningless words. For the first time he feels the witness of David's psalm:

> The heavens are telling the glory of God and the firmament proclaims his handiwork. Day to day pours forth speech and night to night declares knowledge. There is no speech, nor are there words; their voice is not heard, yet their voice goes out through all the earth, and their words to the end of the world. (Psalm 19:1–4)

Davis's book is unique. While some may not be able to accept his theology we cannot argue with his experience of living with Alzheimer's disease.

He warns that the spiritual changes he experiences may not be the last word on this subject. He tells his story out of a context of Christian faith which stands within a long tradition of Christian thinking that links rationality and self-awareness with 'being in the image of God'. In that tradition little emphasis is given to formal liturgy or symbols in worship. The scripture is given more prominence than the sacrament. In such a tradition those suffering failing mental powers must feel very distant from God. I do not know of any record of a person in a tradition where sacrament symbols, colour, formal liturgy and stained glass windows abound who has shared his or her personal spiritual experience of Alzheimer's disease. My observation is that when the brain fails, God, the creator, is known in the human heart and God's presence is felt there. This is so through most of the three stages of the disease.

The fact is that I and many others have heard a number of people with dementia express a spiritual wisdom in the hours just prior to death. Certainly we must learn to develop an understanding of humanness which accords worth and value to affectivity – feeling – if we are to nurture the human spirit of a person with failing mental powers.

What of those who do not claim any religious belief at all? What spiritual changes do they experience and how can we bring nourishment for the spirit, the soul and the heart to them? It is my experience that we must rediscover for them those resources which have always sustained them in life's hard places.

Nurturing spiritual well-being

We have defined the challenges facing the care-giver who desires to bring holistic care, including the spiritual dimension, to those with a primary dementia illness. We have reviewed some of their spiritual changes and losses. I will now share some ways which appear to have been successful in nurturing the human spirit of people with Alzheimer's disease and other primary dementia conditions.

Of course care homes and hospitals for confused older people have always been staffed by some nurse managers who, without fully realising the spiritual significance of what they do, have furnished these places in homely style, providing comfortable seating, arrangements of fresh flowers and attractive pictures to which memory-impaired people may respond and relate. These places have fostered sociability and relatedness with smaller spaces and seating arrangements. Some have developed gardens in which their residents may walk or view from wide, simply-dressed windows. Such enlightened managers provide music which is likely to be of the era in which the residents were young adults. They provide television for specific purposes with programmes like *Songs of Praise* and nature programmes which cue good memories of old, loved and well-known hymns and of animals, birds, flowers and trees. They provide creative and physical activities, visits and walks. All this and more is done, not just to impress relatives looking for a rest home for someone they love, but because they intuitively understand that spiritual care is anchored in the ordinary. It is not reserved for 'church' or the clergyperson's visit.

All staff in the care home and everyone who visits a person in hospital, care home or their own home has the opportunity to nurture spiritual well-being for those unable to do that for themselves. Whenever someone grasps the opportunity to share community, to encourage relatedness, to momentarily reclaim a little identity, or to share some little task of creativity no matter how simple, that person is helping to nurture the spirit and heal and strengthen the soul.

Derek was the young gardener at a recently opened new rest home for people with Alzheimer's disease and related disorders in South Australia. I talked with him about the garden he was developing. He had a good degree in horticulture and a diploma in landscaping. He knew the best way to landscape the site and he certainly knew which plants, flowers and trees would best thrive in the climate. He shared his excitement with me in drawing up his designs and planting plans; he was thrilled with the opportunity to use his recently acquired qualifications. 'But all that', he told me, 'was before the residents began to arrive. Some began to follow me around the embryo garden.'

Within a week he had scrapped all his fine plans. As the residents talked to him about the gardens they had known and loved, and as they bent their old backs and wiggled arthritic hands in the dry red soil he realised that his plans matched the theory of good garden making but might contribute little to the wholeness and well-being of the people who would walk there or admire his work from the windows. Some, he realised with a jolt, might even work in it.

So with much mulching, feeding and watering, lovely roses grew and bloomed in places the experts had advised they never would. Derek had listened and paid attention. He knew that old Mrs B and prim little Miss M loved roses above all other flowers. If he met them in the rose garden he observed that many of the roses cued special memories. One day Mrs B told him how she had filled the house with Dublin Bay and Iceberg each Christmas. Miss M recalled the 'dear wee Cecille Brunner bud' worn in her father's lapel almost every Sunday for church. He noticed that they told the same stories over and over again, as if each were a brand new memory told for the first time. Mr Mac told him to leave the last blooms for hips: 'They're like us, you know, better for seeding.' There was even rhubarb in that garden, and when it was mature and flourishing old Bert, who in his younger days had been second gardener on a large property in Devon, would appear unannounced in the kitchen with a wide armful of thick red rhubarb.

And so Derek's garden, which was no longer just *his* garden, grew like a large patchwork quilt with areas of blue forget-me-nots, purple pansies, red poppies, lavender, white and pink granny-bonnets, love-in-the-mist and tall hollyhocks. All cued many happy memories for residents and staff. Families loved remembering too and visiting ceased to be a strained, awkward experience when the members related with each other and the garden.

Derek had never heard that people's spirits are nurtured in gardens. He did not know that the smell of roses fed their souls. He was unaware that a wide armful of rhubarb would provide Mr Justice T, who had sat severely on the bench for twenty years, with the opportunity to dead-head the stalks. He sat alongside Bert now as they trimmed the bright red stalks so that they looked like strange little Irish leprechauns, with skin-head haircuts sporting defiant bright tufts of rhubarb-green hair.

Spiritual health is nurtured when people experience relationship with their environment, themselves, other people and their God. All four, Derek discovered, are always present in a garden. Derek's skills went beyond those of a fine competent gardener. He listened, observed and intelligently reflected and came to the conclusion that he had control over a resource capable of making a considerable difference to the quality of life for the people for whom the garden existed. To his critics, who had expected a show-standard garden – and conveyed their disappointment – he calmly explained that he was applying the principle of gardening for blind people to gardening for people with brain failure.

He was right. Just as blind people 'saw' the garden through their noses, so 'his' people saw the garden through their feelings as these were resurrected by memories cued about other gardens in other places. In Derek I saw a man who was not religious but who had a deep spiritual awareness, showing kindness and walking humbly with the Creator.

Tools for spiritual well-being

Here are some tools for ministry with people with a primary dementia illness. I shall explain them in that context but they may be used by nurses, care givers and others in their particular relationship with the disabled person. They are:

- principles of communication
- orientation to present reality
- affirmation of feelings
- memory cueing.

Principles of communication

We are social beings made to be in relationship with others. Making relationships and maintaining relationships with others is an important part of our humanity. Human beings are diminished when they remain in isolation. Relationship depends upon communication. Communication is not limited to the oral word – as any monk vowed to silence could confirm. Most people have choices in communication and relationships. The person with Alzheimer's disease and related conditions is largely dependent on the efforts of others to make and maintain relationship.

Content	Early stages	Middle stages	Late stages
Ideas	May drift from topic Difficulty understanding new information Vague Difficulty producing series of relevant sentences	Frequently repeats ideas and forgets topic Talks about past events and trivia with fewer ideas	Unable to produce sequence of related ideas Content irrelevant and bizarre Marked repetition of words and phrases
Words	Vocabulary shrinking Trouble finding right word	Word-finding problems Difficulty naming objects	Poor vocabulary May use jargon Marked naming difficulties
Grammar	Generally correct	Sentences broken up Longer complex sentences not understood	Lack of understanding of many grammatical forms Sentences fragmented
Use	Long-winded but knows when to talk Apathetic – fails to initiate conversation when it would be appropriate Difficulty following humour, sarcasm, non-literal statements May try to correct errors Gestures begin to reduce	Knows when to talk Recognises questions May fail to greet Poor social skills Rarely corrects errors	Generally unaware of surroundings and context Insensitive to others Little relevant language Some mute and some echolalia

Table 3.1: Effects of dementia on communication

Courtesy of L. Ferguson, 24/2/92

In communication theory we talk about a sender, a receiver and the message. The message links the sender and the receiver. Anything which obscures the message is called static. In ministering to people with dementia our task is to eliminate as much static as possible. Lorraine Ferguson, a New Zealander working with people with Alzheimer's disease and related dementia in a London day care centre, provides a chart (Table 3.1) to identify the major communication skills changes at each stage of Alzheimer's disease. Other primary dementia communication changes may not fit this chart. Multi-infarct dementia communication skill, for instance, will be dependent on the number and spacing of the small strokes which may affect speech; these have an immediate effect but may improve in just a few days after the stroke.

The chart above is helpful in guarding care givers from unrealistic expectations of what is possible and probable. Not knowing what is impossible can be a major cause of static. Then care givers fail to communicate for relationship maintenance.

GENERAL PRINCIPLE

- Remember your purpose – relationship building. Doctors and social workers and others whose work necessitates an emphasis on information-seeking communication rather than relationship-building communication have sometimes concluded that, because it is extremely difficult to obtain information from people with dementia, all communication is therefore too difficult to warrant the effort.

- Assume there is capacity for insight. You may be successful where others appear to have failed.

- If you do not understand the person, tell him or her. Ask for the statement to be repeated. If this causes an upset you can try your best guess. Even if you are wrong you have honoured personhood with your honesty.

- Keep your promises. Do not abuse personhood by assuming 'it doesn't matter' or 'she won't remember'.

- Be alert for signs of embarrassment, frustration and anxiety and respond appropriately. Remember, pity is not good enough. If you are a Christian pastor you are there to be the compassion of Christ to this person, not to become anxious because you cannot 'fix it' and make it better. You can be a companion in this person's painful journey for a time and that is far more helpful.

- Regularity and constancy of contact strengthens orientation.

- Most people with Alzheimer's disease are more confused during the late afternoon. As a pastor I find it best to avoid visiting at that time.

SPECIFIC PRINCIPLES

- **Use simple, short sentences.**

- Identify yourself at every visit. You may become 'a familiar friendly' but do not expect to be remembered by name. Introduce yourself by name each time you visit. 'I am...' A name badge is useful with those in the early stages of the disease; if they can read it they will bless you for it. It saves face and preserves dignity.

- Clergy should observe that clerical dress conveys a message and is a way of using all the memory cues at the person's command.

- Address the person by name and try to make and keep eye contact.

- Use the orientation tools of place, day, weather, season, and so on. For example: 'Today is Tuesday... It is sunny... It is springtime... The daffodils are flowering in the park...' and so on.

- Speak slowly and clearly but try not to overdo it to the point of being artificial. Do not raise your voice if you do not get the desired response; only speak louder if the person is hearing impaired and even then be sensitive. Hearing-impaired people are better assisted by being able to see your face – especially your lips – as you speak, rather than by shouting; that only adds to the confusion.

- Wait for a response. Hesitation may be due to a lack of understanding or an inability to frame a prompt reply to what is understood. What may seem to you like an unproductive silence may very well be a hard-work concentration time for the person with dementia.

- Avoid questions if the answer depends on the person remembering facts. Only when you try this will you realise how hard it is to do and how often we all use a question to start a conversation. Remember, your prime purpose is not to elicit information but to build a relationship in which names are of importance.

More specific guidance is given in Appendix 7 and Appendix 8.

NONVERBAL GUIDELINES

- Stand, kneel or sit in front of the person. Of course, it is better to be on the same level but the lack of visitor seating in most rest home lounges makes that difficult. More often than not I find myself on my knees.

- Try to maintain eye contact.

- Use gestures, but meaningfully and not too extravagantly.

- Always check with the staff for any hearing and vision deficits and modify your communication style appropriately. Remember that blindness separates a person from things but impaired hearing separates a person from people so it is more often damaging to spiritual health.

- Learn to control a wheelchair while walking at its side. Try to put yourself, as a confused, memory-impaired person, into a wheelchair and imagine moving into unknown space, not knowing who walks behind you.

- Avoid sudden, quick movements – be calm, slow, flowing in all you do.

The person with Alzheimer's disease is uncertain of the most basic communication tool: speech. Learn to interpret body language and to be aware of your own body language. Touch is important. Holding both hands gently helps to focus the person's attention. A smile really is the shortest distance between two people. My experience is that the most disturbed and noisy person will eventually return a genuine smile.

Orientation to the present reality

Reality orientation is a well-known theory and mode of care which claims to help severely memory-impaired and confused people to organise thinking and remember patterns. This is not what I mean by orientation to the present reality, although I use some of the principles of the theory and find them helpful. The difference is that while I find it can be helpful initially in an encounter to bring the person with Alzheimer's disease into the present reality as it is defined and experienced by most people in the world, I am also ready to respect that this person's reality is different from mine but valid for him or her. It is my responsibility to find a way to reach or communicate with that person in his or her reality. I will not use pressure for the person to stay in my reality.

I would try to bring the impaired person into the reality of the present moment by greeting by name: 'Hello John. I'm Eileen. I'm the minister' (that will be reinforced by the way I am dressed). 'I visit you every Tuesday. Today is Tuesday. We are at Sunnydale Hospital. You live here. I am visiting you, John.' I might then wait for a response before perhaps stating the weather and perhaps the season. That would be how I would begin the pastoral conversation. But it is not a rigid approach; sometimes I may not be able to introduce myself or even make a greeting because the needs of John's reality are urgent.

Affirmation and response to feelings

Early in this ministry I realised that I listen at two levels. At one level I may be hearing a lot of unrelated pain, complaining, grizzling; perhaps a story of:

> working hard all morning in the garden with no one to help me, all alone, work. He said we would go to see Grandpa. He didn't come. I want to go to my grandpa's house. I want to play with the kittens (getting angry now) I'm going to see Grandpa. I'm going. I'm going! (almost shouting).

At one level of listening, what I hear is nonsense. It is a jumble of confused memories. This man is 86 years old and his grandfather has been dead for a very long time. I do not collude with that nor do I deny it. I am paying attention at another level. Behind the confusion what I am hearing in his feelings is more likely to help me to reach meaningfully into his reality. If I can discern that, I can affirm his feelings in his reality. I can be with him in it as a sympathetic friend. Then we are in relationship as two human beings. There is mutuality, too, because at some time I, and most people, have felt as he does now. It is possible to share the pain rather than to 'fix' it from outside.

In Alzheimer's disease we know that it is the recent memory which is lost first. Some of the remote memory remains, even into the most advanced stages of the disease. If we can cue the memory, we are re-minding in order to re-member the person with dementia back into his community or group where his identity is located.

Many years ago the psychologist William James (1950) proposed that a person's sense of identity, which gives moment-by-moment meaning to the pronoun 'I', is dependent on the flow of consciousness of the present (that is, writing this) flowing back to the memory of what I did this morning, yesterday, last week, last month, last year, twenty years ago and more. This gives me the sense of being the same person now as then, in spite of the changes that have taken place around me. When memory functions are lost we lose touch with our own personal reality and history. God (or the source of our spiritual well-being) must then seem terrifyingly far off. No wonder that the first spiritual change experienced by Robert Davis (1989) was fear.

Memory cueing

The good news is that memory can be cued or triggered. Everyone has experienced this and everyone will recognise what it is that cues his or her own memory. Whenever I smell flowering currant I am back in the quad of my old school. I am standing with the rest of the assembled school and the sun is warm on my back. My black woollen stockings itch my legs, the sky is blue and the headmaster's voice is droning on and on. I never think of that time until I smell flowering currant. But when my memory is cued all that is real. I *feel* the sun, I *see* the sky, I *hear* the voice. I am *there*, with all the familiar security of childhood. It is a good feeling. All is well for me in the memory of a safe and happy schoolgirl world.

When we remember an experience from the past, with the raised memory come the feelings associated with the original experience. We know from the work of Brown and Ellor (1981) that the ability to feel and to respond to feelings remains intact in the person with Alzheimer's disease. Those people who care for and minister to people with this disease will find it rewarding to learn as much as possible about the person's memory processes before the disease took over. What cues were most effective in the past for organising information and for remembering? Were they colours, smells, sounds, music, voices, textures? It will take time and patience and a large measure of grace and goodwill of family and friends as well as the commitment of the caregivers and the minister. It is possible.

JIM

In Jim's case the memory cue was smell – the smell of flowers.

I first met Jim when he was in his late seventies and resident in a nursing home since his family could no longer cope with the demands of his Alzheimer's disease type dementia. He was a professional man who had been highly respected in the city and in his church community. When I first started to visit him he was silent. He had not spoken for many months. Sometimes when I spoke to him he would smile sadly but that was all. His family had almost given up visiting. It all seemed to be so unrewarding. The father they knew seemed no longer present. Jim was remote, apparently unreachable until one day, on my way to the nursing home, I visited a parishioner who, as we walked out to my car, picked for me from her garden a little bunch of lily-of-the-valley. I loved it. It had strong memory cues for me.

When I arrived at the nursing home I parked the car and looked hard at that little bunch of such sweet scent and exquisite beauty and I wanted to keep it. But I knew that when I came back to my warm car each little flower would have drooped and withered. So I picked up the flowers and took them with me. I held them close to Jim's face and said, 'Look what I've brought you. Smell them!' And he did. He opened his mouth and the language poured out like water from a broken dam. He told me of the garden he remembered as a boy, of the layout of that garden, the names of the flowers and how much he loved them all. He told me how that garden had always had the power to renew and refresh him. Before my eyes in a few moments he became a different man. He sat up straight. His face was animated. He was alive and enjoying himself.

I never visited Jim after that without a few flowers with a distinctive perfume. They never failed to cue his memory. Once he told me the names of the flowers in his young bride's wedding bouquet. He recalled that special day – his joy in their love, the strong sense of family and friends in the church he had known all his life – in the presence of God whom he knew as creator, the source of his life and well-being.

Of course, I would not be at the bottom of the stairs on my way out before Jim had forgotten me and our conversation. But the good feelings that the resurrection of his memory brought to him remained with him after I had gone, giving him a sense of well-being, identity and belonging.

I told his family of this 'miracle' and they also used the scent of flowers to cue their father's memory. In this way they became 'connected' again. They shared common memories of the past and with those memories all the feelings that were part of each original experience. For them it was a time of healing, a preparation for the separation that his death would eventually bring.

And for Jim, I believe those times of remembering provided the remaining evidence of his identity and a confirmation of his lifelong walk with God.

Jim died about nine months after that first memory-cueing visit. It was a peaceful death. Through the memory cue of the smell of flowers he had been able to talk again with his family. Healing and reconciliation had taken place. He died with a sense of peace and belonging. There is no way of telling, of course, but he could have died in fear and in silence and in isolation from his family. And, worst of all, he could have died separated in his own dementia experience from the source of his spiritual well-being, his creator God who nourished his spirit and gave him such joy and pleasure in the flowers he loved.

CHARLOTTE

Charlotte was born in 1910. From a very early age high academic expectations were placed on her. Clearly she was successful. Her accomplishments are impressive when one recalls her age and gender. She won a university scholarship and graduated with MA Honours, majoring in English literature. She was a skilled and nationally recognised potter. She held high office in her women's service club. For many years she was senior mistress of a large school.

Charlotte never married. Her work and hobbies and her intellectual pursuits gave her life meaning and purpose. She had been raised in the church, had a strong intellectual interest in religion, loved the scriptures and, one suspects, regarded God as a stern arbitrator of human morality and judge of individual deservingness.

In 1989 Charlotte was admitted to hospital for assessment. She was diagnosed as suffering a dementia illness, almost certainly Alzheimer's disease. The loss of the ability to reason, to think, to organise and remember was, for this lady, an immeasurable loss.

Eventually she was admitted to a care home and when I first met her she was a little curled-up form sitting forlornly on the terrace, waiting – waiting for someone who never came. She mixed with no one. I introduced myself as the Methodist minister and a fellow schoolteacher. I was accepted and we talked. She wafted in and out of confusion and the present reality. She referred to the other residents as pupils 'not worth wasting your time with, dear. Definitely, definitely not scholarship material!'. In an effort to cue her memory and deal with the reality behind her confusion I made a stab in the dark and said, 'Well, Charlotte, you have an MA degree in English literature. You must have a favourite poet.' It was a statement, not a question.

Immediately she exclaimed, 'Oh, yes. Shakespeare... She straightened up from a curled-over foetal position. Her whole body was in joyful anticipation. She was in command. She opened her mouth and out flowed Portia's beautiful mercy speech from *The Merchant of Venice*:

> the quality of mercy is not strain'd,
> It droppeth as the gentle rain from heaven
> Upon the place beneath: it is twice bless'd;

Here she faltered a little and I came in:

> It blesseth him that gives and him that takes:

'Ah,' she said:

> 'Tis mightiest in the mightiest; it becomes
> The throned monarch better than his crown;
> His sceptre shows the force of temporal power,
> The attribute to awe and majesty,
> Wherein doth sit the dread and fear of kings;
> But mercy is above this sceptred sway,
> It is enthroned in the hearts of kings.

Once again she faltered and once again I helped her:

> It is an attribute...

And in she came again:

> ...to God himself,
> And earthly power doth then show likest God's
> When mercy seasons justice.

We finished that last line together, heads back, loving the music in the words and laughing in sheer delight. Charlotte's face was shining and her eyes were bright and alert. She clasped my arm and we laughed into each other's eyes as we recited. We were intimately related in that sharing moment.

This loved and remembered poetry was brief evidence of her identity. She was whole. There was a long pause and then, very firmly, she said, 'Oh, my goodness, that was good... The music of my soul.' She smiled, breathing deeply, and after a number of seconds, perhaps even minutes, she whispered, 'I love that tree.' It was a very beautiful maple. 'I'm glad it is there for you,' I answered gently. Still smiling softly and still looking at the tree, she wafted again into confusion. 'They're a poor lot, you know. Definitely not scholarship material.'

What nourishes spiritual well-being? I have come to see that the answer is very individual. For Charlotte I believe it is words: noble words, beautiful poetry. Shakespeare, Browning, Milton and Blake are poets whose work she can still recite if the memory is cued for her. She remembers long passages of scripture also. All this language, noble language, language that empties from the mouth as a sacrament to enter the ears to speak to the heart, to feed the human spirit. It is life-giving and as essential to her spiritual well-being as an icon, a crucifix, a psalm, a prayer, a symphony, the sacred writings or a silent mountain are for others.

I have chosen to share Jim's and Charlotte's stories to illustrate the changes in people's lives when time is taken to cue the memory and to meet the reality of feelings behind the confusion and isolation. For Jim this meant healing, peace, belonging and reconciliation in the final days of his life. For Charlotte it meant a sense of identity, a greater sociability, a confidence in her new home, a warmth and kindness with others and a peace within herself that was not evident when we first met.

When spiritual well-being is integrated into physical and psychosocial needs the pastor, and all those with spiritual awareness who have been trained to communicate effectively, can make a significant contribution towards the total well-being of the person with dementia.

Some thoughts for care givers

Already I have tried to emphasise the wholeness of the care-giver's role. The spiritual is a vital ingredient of all of life. The needs of the human spirit do not wait until priest or presbyter comes with prayers, hymns, holy words and sacrament, although these will be important resources for people of faith. The care giver who showers a resident with respect for the human body, who is attentive to the vulnerability of the human psyche and aware of the needs of the human spirit is providing spiritual care. So are the cook and kitchen staff when food is prepared with respect for the gifts of the earth and presented to please the eye and nose as well as nourish the body.

Resources

Wherever there is beauty the human spirit is uplifted. Here are some valuable resources in the provision of holistic care:

- well-chosen pictures, hung where they can be enjoyed and at a height where they can be easily seen from a sitting position

- music, perhaps of popular songs of an earlier era in the residents' life – old-time dance music and well-known hymns

- flowers, with consideration for scent, colour and form. Those who wish to share a little of the burden of the care giver at home could change a bad day to joy if flowers were brought to cheer. They should not be left in a bunch but arranged in water. Believe it or not, a bunch of flowers out of water can become a minor nightmare to the 'stretched' care giver who is very much behind with the day

- poetry, read aloud, for those who have a lifelong appreciation. I have seen a group of confused memory-impaired residents delighted with Pam Ayers's verse and others obviously 'in touch' listening to recordings of some of Stanley Holloway's monologues about Albert, who was swallowed by the lion or 'Sam, Sam, pick up tha' musket'. These and other recitations cue memories for many whose sole Saturday night entertainment was radio.

I am wary of anything that tempts us to relate to confused older people as we would to children. But I have observed an activities organiser and a small group of people with early second-stage Alzheimer's disease having the time of their lives reciting and singing nursery rhymes. The staff person started the rhyme: 'Humpty Dumpty sat...' and the voices started to join in: '...on a wall. Humpty Dumpty...'. Then with a burst of recovered memory almost everyone joined in for 'had a great fall'. 'One, two, buckle my shoe,' with hand claps was a favourite. This activity seemed to provide fun without threat. When one person forgot someone else remembered and so they carried each other along.

All my life I have found pleasure in the simple verse of A.A. Milne. 'The Little Black Hen' (Milne 1927) is a favourite and I've read it so many times to receptive children I know it off by heart. If one day I have to journey into forgetfulness and confusion I hope someone will say to me 'Berryman and Baxter, Prettiboy and Penn'. I know I shall burst in then with 'And old Farmer Middleton are five big men, and all of them were after the little Black Hen'.

Once, sitting in isolating, sad, desperate silence with an old gentleman well advanced into second-stage Alzheimer's disease, I started to sing softly a school playground song of my own experience: 'Will you come to Abyssinia, will you come, Will you come to Abyssinia, will you come?' To my utter and delighted surprise it worked. Recognition warmed his eyes and he joined me in a very loud voice, 'Mussolini will be there, shooting peanuts in the air, will you come...' As we finished he grabbed my hand, held it and laughed and laughed.

Now you could be thinking 'crazy woman!'. No matter, I have learned to be glad for opportunities to be a bit of a clown for God. I know that one of the sweetest, most normalising experiences any of us can have is that of sharing joy. It is of little significance that this sharing was over a piece of warmongering playground doggerel. Briefly we had entered each other's world, each with a crowd of associated memories. For me, sunshine, a playground filled with the high-pitched noise of many happy, playing children and I am part of it all. For the old man beside me? Who knows? It does not matter. Briefly, precious intimacy is experienced. That is important for the health of the human spirit and God is surely in it.

The natural environment: trees, sky, sea, lakes and river

I have a memory which illustrates the power of the outdoor environment to heal the spirit even in a large city. In Manchester, Janet, the nursing sister in charge of November Ward, and the chaplain shared a very special experience with me. May was an elderly woman who had been a resident of the ward for five years. Gradually during that time her dementia illness had brought her to almost total silence. She did not appear to be unhappy but she was not sociable and liked sitting alone by the upstairs window. About six months before my visit she had been diagnosed with a fast-growing inoperable cancer. Although pain control was successful and May could not remember the cancer she appeared to be very depressed. Certainly she had changed from the quiet co-operative little woman that staff had always known. She cried often, wringing her hands in seeming anguish. Janet and her staff and the chaplain wanted her dying to be painless and peaceful but first they wanted her to live until she died. While she suffered very little physical discomfort it was obvious that she had little peace. Staff who had responsibility for her care conferred with Janet and the chaplain to plan for her spiritual care during these final weeks.

They knew that she was not a religious woman. She had never indicated any interest in the regular chapel services of worship, although staff had observed her quiet pleasure in all growing things that came into the third-floor ward. Although she rarely approached any small children or babies of visiting families she watched and smiled. The questions they all wanted answered and to which they were prepared to give time, energy and intelligence were: what resources has May always used to nourish her spirit?; is she still in touch with these resources?; can we identify these?; can we find ways to help her access them?

It was decided to have a family consultation to discuss these matters. Janet and the chaplain met with May's daughters. Could they remember what had sustained their mother when life was particularly hard for her? Eventually as they chatted and shared together one of the daughters remembered her mother's passionate love of trees. They recalled and shared their memories of a dark period of the War. Their father was on active service abroad. There had been no mail for weeks and rumours abounded. The city was suffering heavy bombing night after night. A bomb had fallen in their street and a friend's toddler was wounded and then died. Janet said it was very, very hard for them and there were tears as these painful memories, suppressed seemingly for so long, were given expression and articulated. Each woman recalled her bewilderment and fear as their mother became more and more silent and withdrawn.

The chaplain and Janet sympathetically wondered aloud how a young mother in such circumstances had found strength to come through to meaning and purpose. The daughters thought they knew. Every day, they said, she went to the park alone and walked and walked under the oaks, elms, beech and sycamore trees. She had been raised in a small village. 'Our mother loved trees, grass and space,' they said. Once, not long after the War, she had talked to them of the little child's death. The eldest daughter had always remembered the seemingly strange thing she had told them of that time: 'The trees gave me their strength'.

On the next fine day May was lovingly wrapped warmly, put in a wheelchair, and a nurse and a care giver pushed her to the nearest park. Once there they placed the chair under the trees and withdrew a little way. After a few minutes May straightened her head and shoulders, looked up and exposed her face which she cupped as if bathing it in the cool, fresh air. Many months had passed since this woman had been outside the hospital. Something as basic and life-giving as the fresh air on her skin was now a luxury seldom experienced. Her body seemed relaxed, although expectant too, as she lifted her eyes to the pattern of branches, leaves and grey sky above her. I was told that she became almost motionless as although her whole self was in the process of being concentrated into the grass, the trees, the air and the sky. Once, her eyes caught the quick movement of a sparrow and followed it as it rose to branches high above her. And although tears washed her cheeks she gave the impression of gentle beauty and profound peace. She did not speak – it was always difficult for her to put words together.

After a reasonable time, her care givers approached and wheeled her back to the hospital. That evening, as her nurse settled her in bed and said goodnight, May whispered, 'I tasted the sky. God held me up'. May became less restless, less seemingly angry and anxious. She stopped crying and one nurse said, 'It was like she was hugging close to herself a sweet, sweet secret. We all felt happy for her.' Within the week May died. As far as anyone knew her words to her bedtime nurse on the night of the day they had taken her to the park were her last.

This story illustrates how richly the human spirit can be nourished by God's self-revelation in all creation. Spirituality may have little or nothing to do with 'churchiness'. Sister Janet and the chaplain of November Ward understood very well what had 'resourced' May towards a good and peaceful dying. She had been reconnected to the environment she had always found to be her sustaining help in the face of tragedy and undeserved suffering. She was cued into meaningful relationship with the natural environment, the creator God, herself and at least one other person, her night nurse. May was not a religious person but in her last days her care givers had found a way, essentially spiritual, to ease her death with hope and peace.

Others will almost certainly recall similar experiences when, in the presence of deeply felt natural beauty, they have known inner-connectedness and a sharp, almost painful but sweet awareness of every detail of a leaf, a flower, a blade of grass or even a resting butterfly. This sense may be so strong that there may be a need to embrace a tree, cradle a little snowdrop, speak to the mountain or listen to the secrets of a seashell to celebrate the overwhelming sense of belonging, of being intimately related, a meaningful part of the whole of creation. At such times something very precious stirs within us, an exquisite yearning so powerful we turn right around, reaching out to the eternal mystery who is the source of all that is, as distant as the farthest star, as close as our own breath. Poets, artists, musicians and prophets are often closely in tune with such experiences, so spiritually aware that they may spend a lifetime trying adequately to express the mystery. The world may pronounce some of them mad, many may ignore them and some, becoming anxious about the spark that fires their passion, would have them put away. Only the children and the childlike understand and love them.

Acceptance

This means not trying to change people just because they have different views, tastes, cultural values, likes and dislikes from ourselves. It means respecting people because each person is a unique human being. Acceptance is being reconciled to our own mortality. Alzheimer's disease is, after all, part of being human until the good intention of the creator God, source of all that is, lover of the least, is established on the earth in all its promised fullness. Aligning ourselves with that holy intention, which is already accomplished and yet also not here, is to bring its fullness closer.

Acceptance means respecting others' beliefs. It means sharing the losses and pains of this destructive disease with those who walk the journey. It means also accepting our own physical limitations and forgiving ourselves for the mistakes we make.

Listening

Care givers offer not only their physical presence but also their receptivity, their openness and their genuine attention. It can also mean, especially for the home care giver, knowing when to stop listening and seek one's own inner place of stillness and quiet. There must be space for absence as well as presence.

Spiritual well-being and administration

Information collected at admission for the purposes of care management for individual residents should include these details which could be crucial in the provision of spiritual and religious care.

SPIRITUAL

If the family have been able to prepare a life history of the confused and memory-impaired person, this can be a very worthwhile resource for professional care givers in alerting them to possible memory cues, names, hobbies, skills, world view, particular concerns, interests and involvement as well as preferences and dislikes. Most important will be to identify those things that have given strength, purpose and meaning to their lives.

Some families will have little interest in such a resource or have few of the skills necessary for its compilation. To assist them and to streamline the task it is as well to have prepared an admission form beforehand. This can be given to a responsible family person to fill in and return. But I favour the home manager and family doing this together. A spouse, a daughter, son or another close relative leaving a loved person in a nursing home needs this opportunity to build their confidence in the person responsible for care. This is a time also to talk about the family's continuing role in the loved one's care. Most families will need a lot of help with communicating in the new environment. Relationship is an important component of spiritual well-being. It is worth spending time to teach families how to do this well.

RELIGIOUS

The following information is necessary (a prepared question-and-answer document is a good way to get this from families):

- religion (Muslim, Christian, etc.)
- faith tradition (if Christian, Roman Catholic, Baptist, etc.)
- name, contact telephone number and postal address of clergyperson or other religious person to contact if necessary in an emergency for example, near-death, spiritual or religious difficulty. Parish clergy often lose contact with an elderly confused parishioner at this time because family have not thought to advise them.

It can be very helpful to send a routine card to clergy. When I have suggested this I have often been surprised by the manager's reply: 'Oh, I've never written to a clergyman. I wouldn't know how.' It must be remembered with respect and sensitivity that people who do not go to church are aware that church culture exists. Most want to be courteous and respectful of it but are quite uncertain how to proceed. I offer the following:

The Minister/Pastor/Elder
(or other religious leader)

Dear (name)

Recently Mr/Mrs/Mrs_____ has come to live in our care home. Her/his family has named you as his/her minister/pastor/leader/priest/elder.

We aim to provide holistic care for our residents and consider the spiritual and religious dimensions of care to be essential for the resident's quality of life and well-being.

May we ask that you confirm with us your readiness to be responsible for the provision of_____'s religious needs and to assist us in the provision of spiritual well-being for him/her.

We would be very pleased to welcome you as a valued associate and ask you to make yourself known to us in our reception area. We will do all we can to assist you. This is important and urgent. We appreciate in anticipation your early response.

Yours sincerely

Home Manager

Address and phone number

If the care home provides a return reply card and self-addressed envelope a reply will be more certain.

More suggestions

- Have a quiet room with perhaps one or two religious symbols, for example, a cross or pictures which, although perhaps not specifically religious, have a spiritual significance. Provide staff or volunteers who can accompany a resident there for stillness and quietness. This room may also house a cassette machine or CD player so that suitable soft music could provide a soothing, peaceful background. Numerous uses would be found for such a room. Alternatively this could be furnished as a small ecumenical chapel.

- Provide for services of Christian worship. Do not take for granted that all clergy or lay worship leaders will know very much about the intellectual limitations and possibilities of residents or will offer worship relevant to the needs and abilities of people with Alzheimer's disease and related dementias.

It would not be right to interfere in any clergyperson's pastoral visits without valid cause for anxiety over the resident's safety. However, nursing home management has the responsibility of ascertaining the professional competence of any person contributing to total care. I have witnessed some worship which has been totally unsuitable and, although no doubt well-intentioned, was actually abusive of the residents. Long wordy evangelical sermons are not appropriate in these circumstances. The first intention can never be to 'win people for Christ'. Rather it is to recognise each person as precious to, and loved by, the one who created each of us and to affirm this in every possible way.

Not all parish clergy are capable of adapting ordinary modes of worship to the needs of people with a dementia illness. Generally they know very little about dementia. Unless care home management is willing to employ trained chaplains, worship will only be available with the goodwill of local parish clergy. In my considered view and experience, a relationship of mutual accountability is essential. Worship leaders, lay and clerical, need to seek training for this aspect of ministry which can only become a greater and more demanding component of Christian ministry as the aged population increases.

At the same time care home management legally carry the responsibility for the provision of good quality care and safety of their residents. The management needs to be capable of assessing the professional competence of all those providing a necessary service to residents, for example, physiotherapists, chiropodists, hairdressers and many others including the clergyperson. Traditionally, local clergy have offered services to care homes as an extension of the work they do for their congregations and communities as part of their church's mission. Christian congregations – and other religious communities – have carried the cost of that ministry themselves. However, the growing number of care homes in parishes and our developing understanding of the needs of people with dementia, together with the greatly increasing older population generally, have dramatically changed the balance between the people who need service and care and those with energy and resources to provide it.

Forms of community chaplaincy are an important need as the State embraces and implements an ideology of community care. The situation presents an urgent dilemma for the Christian community. The care home industry should consider this sympathetically. Both parties must seek a solution in the spirit of the one who continually sought out those who suffered and were marginalised by the politically and religiously powerful of his day and had compassion on them. For the rest it is to be hoped that as much fervour and speed is brought to the rights of old people with failing mental powers as the human rights movement is bringing to our society's other marginalised groups, such as indigenous people or the gay community.

Care home management could assist clergy who conduct worship in dementia care homes by providing a clergy information pack or leaflet including at least the following:

- names of staff
- who to approach for information
- names of residents and brief personal information about new residents
- names of those who have died since the last visit – the worship leader may wish to acknowledge the death, give thanks for the person's life and pray for all those personally affected, including the staff, who often need recognition of their grief
- name of staff member to be informed if the worship leader is unexpectedly unable to lead worship at the scheduled time
- a commitment to inform the clergyperson of any information which might assist. (On one occasion I arrived as usual to lead worship only to find that most of the residents had gone out on a picnic!)
- routines for fire drill
- anything else the manager might consider important and useful, for example, where the staff toilet is located.

All this should be discussed and mutual agreement reached before the commitment to lead worship or provide pastoral care is finalised.

Other responsibilities of the management include:

- contracting to have the worship space ready and residents assembled for when the worship leader arrives
- consulting records for those who will attend. Do not leave it to staff to ask residents, 'Do you want to go to church?' They would not do that about meal-times. You know that many of your residents are unable to cope with questions. Your records should tell you who would wish to go to church. So your approach would be a positive invitation: 'Mr Johnston, the minister/priest is coming for church today. You go to church. You used to go to St Ninian's. Come with me; we'll go together.'
- not leaving the worship leader alone with a lounge full of residents while leading worship. This is not an opportunity for staff to take a break; at least some should be present to deal with any emergency and if they sit by particular residents to assist them that is also part of their caring role.

Some encouragement for those caring at home

Here are some suggestions for those who give care in family homes.

- Help your loved one to continue usual devotional and worship patterns for as long as possible.

- If your loved one is in the early stages of the disease it may be possible to discuss together some of the changes that will undoubtedly come. Now is the time to make important decisions together. Death is probably many years down the track but the ability to discuss that together will, in quite a short time, be stolen from your loved one. You may wish to plan the funeral service, both your sick partner's or relative's and your own. Some will almost certainly find that too difficult, but for those for whom it is important this preparation can be therapeutic and liberating.

- Confide in your minister. Explain what you need from the faith family to help you support your loved one's spiritual well-being and religious practice. Expect to receive it without guilt.

- Ask for the sacrament of communion to be brought to your loved one regularly if this conforms to his or her preferred worship pattern. If it is comfortable for you both, ask a friend to join you in this. Do all you can to cue your loved one's memory into the communion.

- Remember that the Holy Spirit ministers at all times and, if a particular devotional act does not seem to go well, leave it for a time.

- Ask your church family for a support group and be prepared to tell people what help you need. Now is the time to learn the spiritual discipline of gracious receiving without resentment and guilt.

- If it helps you to join the church family at worship ask for someone to sit with your loved one so that you can attend at least every month or six weeks.

- Use recorded music and helpful television or video programmes such as *Songs of Praise.*

- Try to enjoy the outdoors together. Visit the park, botanical gardens, beach and river. Pick the daisies. Smell the flowers. Go swimming together for as long as that is practical. Dance and sing.

- You may like to use the prayer 'Jesus, have mercy' silently over and over in the heart. When caring for my mother I found great comfort and release from tension and tiredness in this. Sometimes my mother would catch me forming the prayer on my lips and would say it herself; very often it seemed to calm her and if I offered it when she was in the endless turning-out of cupboards and drawers stage it would slow her down for a time and she became less frantic. Once as I formed the prayer my little mother caught the first word and exclaimed: 'Jesus! Well, he's not doing much for me today!' What release of tension that provided.

- Enjoy laughter. We often fed the ducks because they always made my mother laugh. And her laughter gifted itself to me so that we laughed together.

- Garden together for as long as your loved one enjoys it.

- Try to find ways to cue the memory and remember together.

- Keep married love physical for as long as that is pleasurable to you both.

- Use therapeutic massage. Aromatic oils can be recommended for use with partners and spouses of people with a dementia illness. We know that being in relationship with another person is an important spiritual resource. Touching is a way of relating when words fail.

- Try to ground your own strong feelings (for example, anger, despair, impatience, etc.) in some kind of action: walking, gardening, using an exercise bike or punch bag.

- Talk it over with someone qualified to understand. If you were employed to do this caring work your contract would almost certainly include provision for professional support and supervision.

- Remember that you will experience grief as your loved one's reality becomes more and more distant from your own. There is nothing static about loss which is more a process than an event or a state. When someone you love and cherish is slowly but relentlessly leaving you, the experience of loss is open at both ends: from the present into the past and from the present into the unknown future. Some people daily losing a partner to dementia not only will experience present pain but will also relive the feelings of old griefs. They cannot help but look into a future which looms bleak and lonely for months and years stretching out before them.

It is wise to try to remember that human beings cannot bear unremitting emotional pain and distress. You may find that you 'switch off' and buffer yourself against it. This is normal: you may contemplate and look steadily at your own and your partner's situation and then look quickly away. You may talk of the reality of your losses and try to get yourself and your life in order and then begin to talk as if all will be as it used to be by the end of summer or whatever. That is normal, too.

You may find yourself oscillating between relaxed chatting – even making a joke of what is happening in your life and sharing the absurd episodes of caring – and shaking and trembling disclosure of new agony and emotional tearing apart of your whole being. This is the time to recover or bring out your own spiritual and religious resources and certainties.

Perhaps hardest of all is the fact that anger is an emotion others tend to back away from. Anger frightens many people but is a large portion of grief. It must be grounded and expressed, but few people understand the process of grieving and that expressing anger may be a very large part of that process. If you spill this out in some situations it may not be understood and friends may desert you just at the time you need them most. A good pastor or a wise friend will recognise this and be available as a place of acceptance.

This suffering is the family care giver's spiritual 'dark night of the soul'. There is no way out; you have to go through it. Beware of those who offer to fix your pain. If you can stay with your suffering while having compassion on yourself you will find that the extent of your compassion for others expands. Then you are no longer alone but discover, by grace, a way of living together so that the mystery, the meaning and purpose of life, are revealed. It takes time and effort, but in the end there is a quiet, joyful solidarity with all humanity.

Summary and conclusions

There is a spiritual dimension to every life. Attention to this dimension is nothing more than acknowledging the full humanity of every person. Dementia illness is a condition of the human brain which does not mean that the whole human being is diseased; the human spirit should be recognised by trained and aware care givers and nourished to provide for a better quality of life. We have described the difference between spiritual and religious in this chapter and identified the essential factors in the provision of spiritual well-being from an understanding which arises out of a wide spectrum of different people. Certainly I have no doubts that the ordinary person is aware that he or she is more than body, brain and breath, whatever he may call that 'something more'.

The practice of religion may be an important resource in meeting spiritual needs and concerns. It is the task of the faith community to make the consolations of religion available to its members who suffer Alzheimer's disease and other related dementia illnesses. I cannot speak for other world faith communities. My own religious experience and spirituality is Christian. With all my heart and intellectual powers I affirm the work of caring being done by so many individual Christian people. The institutional Church, as one would expect, is slower to embrace the implications of an ageing population, dementia, and the obligation which I believe the Christian community is given to include old, confused and memory-impaired people into its life and mission.

That the Church has been slow to honour this obligation is excused by church leaders with an explanation about money – not enough of it. Much hard work in terms of advocacy and education, faith, prayer and plain, focused, clear thinking is required.

The next two chapters are an attempt to share ways by which some spiritual health may be taken to those who cannot remember, think or reason.

4

Worship for People with Alzheimer's Disease and Related Dementias

Let us come into his presence with thanksgiving; let us make a joyful noise to him with songs of praise. (Psalm 95:2)

Most people with Alzheimer's disease and related disorders are denied opportunities for worship. My hope is that this chapter will be a contribution towards changing that. I am convinced that in almost every instance the situation is one more of ignorance than indifference.

When the Church's Ministry to Elderly Confused People was first launched in my city a number of private hospitals and rest home staff contacted me expressing interest and appreciation. They were pleased with the Church's formal commitment to the spiritual health of older people with a dementia illness. It is true that some pastors, lay and ordained, do faithfully visit people in care homes. They might lead a conventional service of worship too. But often almost nothing is done to make that service relevant to those with diminishing powers of remembering, thinking and reasoning. Even fewer attempts are made to meet pastoral needs of a spiritual nature. When church leaders have thought about people with dementia they have identified a health problem and their response has been one of compassionate concern for the physical rather than the spiritual needs of such people.

In many instances care homes have been built and staffed with little or no thought for the spiritual dimension of care. Little money is available for chaplaincy and a modest ecumenical chapel is declared a luxury. Often there is not even a quiet room where people can sit in the stillness of a presence and pray or just 'be'. There is a need for a space which affirms residents in their understanding that they are more than body, brain and breath. No architect, surely, would omit a kitchen or dining-room from a planned care home on the grounds that the patients would be adequately nourished by helping themselves as best as their abilities allowed to snack food left haphazardly around the home. If people are not to suffer malnutrition, catering must be intentional. It is the same for spiritual nourishment. Physical, social, psychological and spiritual needs of patients and residents should be reflected in the building plans of hospitals and care homes.

The extent of the neglect of the spiritual dimension of care for people with dementia is observed in *Ageing* (1990), a report prepared by the Church of England Board of Social Responsibility. This document reports that in both its theology and practice, with the exception perhaps of chaplaincy in psychiatric wards, the church has excluded people with dementia. And we might note that, with the closing of many psychiatric wards and the placement of people with serious dementias into private care homes in the community, even this exception is no longer valid.

Of course there has always existed a small body of individual pastors who have struggled with the theology that has excluded some from worship. They have tackled the enormous challenges of leading relevant worship for confused and severely memory-impaired people so that their spiritual well-being might be nurtured. Such pastors, in my observation, are usually ministers and priests in those Christian traditions which are sacrament-centred and which have also a long tradition of religious orders in the lives of their communions. A heritage of this kind provides for a valuing of silence, solitude, order, 'being', symbol, ritual and the priestly tasks. It is more difficult for some of the reformed traditions whose strength (and weakness) may be attributed to the primacy ascribed to the word – the read word of scripture, the preached word of the sermon, the reasoning word in discussion and careful consensus making. There are also the less thoughtful and often shallow words of endless committee meetings when not a few are dying for a word of life.

Happily there are small signs of change, and a growing desire for a more concentrated and ordered mode of spiritual rehabilitation or renewal is evident among people of some of the more word-centred reformed church traditions. There are those who are seeking out silent and directed retreats and spiritual direction. Some few are even adopting the practice of living by a simple rule of life.

To do so is, for my own Methodist people at least, a returning to our roots. The systematic ordering of personal lives under God is surely one of the most recognized marks of the early Methodists. The roots of this intentional ordering of life under God's spirit grounded themselves deep into the principles by which, for instance, Susanna Wesley (mother of John and Charles) ordered the religious life of her household. They are grounded even deeper still in the life of the great religious orders of the pre-Reformation Church in England. I am convinced that a reclaiming of all that is best of this strong strand of Christian spirituality is essential to an understanding of a mode of ministry which nurtures spiritual growth among our people. Most of all it is essential for the spiritual health and well-being of those with failing cognitive abilities.

A deeply reflective manner of living provides for the spiritual awareness that can accept with sympathetic understanding the chaos and sense of lostness and abandonment that is experienced by people with dementia. These losses are so much worse when the cognitively disabled person has become separated from the worship of his or her church for this is possibly accompanied by a sense of separation from the love of God. We know that the Hebrew people of Ancient Israel experienced identity as they lived in community. The worship acceptable to God emanated from the collective life of the people. Jesus had a special concern for those whose disabilities excluded them from the life of the community. His healing was always to re-integrate, that is, re-member them into the community to which they belonged.

That people with Alzheimer's disease and related disorders are very often denied opportunities to worship as a part of the gathered people of God is a grave scandal. We must acknowledge this and commit ourselves to finding ways to include such people in the life and worship of the Church. We will not do this out of our charity but because it is their right, won for them by Christ's defeat of the powers of chaos and darkness and the glorious reality of his living presence among us. We may well discover a paradox, finding that we are blessed by these 'little ones' who are always close to the loving heart of Jesus.

> She lived life out of a wheelchair,
> Barely hearing, almost blind.
> At worship today
> Christ's supper was offered to her,
> But she thought the plate of broken bread
> Was the offering plate.
> Bewildered, she said, a bit too loud,
> 'I don't have anything to give.'
> Poor woman, they thought.

Not so.

Through any disorientation we have everything
In Christ, who offers his life for us.
Through our deafness he hears for us
Through our blindness he sees for us;
Through our trembling hands he will
Take the bread and cup for us.

We hear Christ's words
Let not your heart be troubled;
I will hold it,
I will feed you.
I will drink the cup for you
I will be your world.
Oh, to be so poor. (Guffey 1991)

We have often been told that all worship should be relevant to the particular situation of the congregation. Such a precept, although wise and true, presents a stern challenge to those who lead worship for people with Alzheimer's disease and similar disorders. Worship leaders will need to use a mode of worship which is relevant to the particular needs of those who are progressively losing the ability to think, to reason and to remember. That there is much more to learn is beyond doubt and it is my hope that, as more people begin to include the needs of people with dementia in the worship plans of the parish, care home or hospital, a network of people-sharing resources will develop. In a small way this has already begun. The work of the Church's Ministry to Elderly Confused People in New Zealand was mentioned at the United Nations Conference of Women in Beijing, China in 1995 through the prompting of a woman in Manchester. The internet is also proving a valuable means of sharing resources.

In this chapter and the associated appendixes I will offer my own experience and some worship modes and resources which I have found to be successful in providing worship that can enrich and sustain the spiritual health and well-being of older people with failing mental powers. It is my hope that these will encourage others to write liturgies relevant to people with Alzheimer's disease and to share them more widely.

Here we must note that each person's experience of Alzheimer's disease is different from everyone else's. It is not possible to claim with absolute accuracy the exact point of any individual's journey through the disease. We can only approximate for the purposes of talking and writing about it. Not every person is likely to experience all the symptoms of any one stage and no two people will progress through the stages at the same rate. With these cautions in mind let us now look at various modes and resources.

Worship needs in the first stage

The first stage of Alzheimer's disease is what Professor Riesberg (1983) calls the 'forgetfulness stage'. People at this stage will mostly still be living in their own homes, some alone, some with a family care giver, often with an aged spouse. Many will be able to continue attending church services.

Rev. Robert Davis (1989), who as we have noted received the diagnosis of very early stage Alzheimer's disease while in his very early fifties, wrote: 'Suddenly I stand out in the worship service, silent and continually confused... I can no longer be spiritually fed by the sermon... It sends my mind whirling in a jumble of twisted unconnected ideas' (p.91).

E's experience was different. It seems that so central was the Church's worship and fellowship to her life that now, in her forgetfulness and confusion, she wanted to be in church every day. Although she was 80 years old she walked to her church almost every day. Suddenly she would notice (or sense) the time, put on her jacket, look for her collection envelope and her purse, and be out of the gate and purposefully on her way. Her faith tradition has no experience of the church as a place of holy presence and private prayer. Six days out of seven E encountered a closed and locked church. However, she was usually noticed by the church secretary who chatted a while, made her a cup of tea and kindly turned her homeward. Some days she laughed at her 'silly mistake' and on others she was observed to be wistfully sad and puzzled.

Never was E made to feel foolish or unwelcome or even unexpected. The women of her church group understood very little of Alzheimer's disease but they knew E. They met her always as a valued person, the friend they had worked with for church fundraising fairs, the friend with whom they had served countless cups of tea at innumerable church gatherings, the friend with whom they had worshipped and prayed, the friend they knew to be true and caring in times of trouble and sickness. They received E as a person, changed – but the same.

I met K at our ecumenical public service of worship which I lead for people with Alzheimer's disease, their families, friends and care givers. This service marks the beginning of Alzheimer's Awareness Week in our city. So normal was he in appearance and manner that had he not told me I might not have known that recently he had been diagnosed as having early first-stage Alzheimer's disease. K was a Christian who had practised his faith and attended worship from youth to middle age when, for no particular reason, he stopped going to church although he continued in irregular prayers and private devotions.

Now, understanding the diagnosis of Alzheimer's disease and the prognosis of increasing memory loss and confusion, he had responded to an invitation to this service and was able to tell me that he had been comforted and encouraged by the knowledge that such a communion of worship was possible for people very much further on in their journey into the disease than he was.

> I need to know that now. I need to know, now, that when I can no longer remember God or even know who I am, others will remind me and gather me into my place in the Church. It is important for me to know that now. Today has been good news for me.

This conversation reminds me of the importance of early diagnosis, not only because symptoms may be due to some treatable condition and much agony easily dispelled but also because at an early stage of the disease the person can do much to help with his or her future care. There are people who tell me that should they be struck down with Alzheimer's disease there is no way they would want to be told. No doubt there are people for whom that would be to their good, and such a view must be respected and accepted. I can only report the conversation with K and the conclusions I have reached out of my observation of the acute anxiety felt by those who may be in the early stages of Alzheimer's disease and who definitely know that something is dreadfully amiss. Knowledge is always power.

People in the early stages of this devastating disease need to know that the priest or pastor understands what lies ahead for them. They need assurance that the Church will not abandon them. If they can be reassured that there are ministers with understanding and the appropriate skills to provide relevant pastoral care and worship opportunities, they can begin to help themselves. They can make necessary business and financial decisions and arrangements for the well-being of their families. A person diagnosed in the early stages has time to right broken relationships and to give and receive forgiveness. There is time to tell spouse and children they are loved and appreciated, no matter what changes are ahead. There is a need for a short and simple ritual which allows the sufferer in the presence of his loved ones to put himself and those he loves under the mercy and protection of a loving God who never forgets his people. All this is likely to ensure strong emotional and spiritual health.

Such preparation is possible also for people who do not practise religion but nevertheless understand that they are spiritual as well as physical, emotional and social beings.

If they have been regular worshippers in the past, most people in an early stage of Alzheimer's disease will wish to remain in their own worshipping congregation for as long as they – and their care givers and others – find that helpful and reasonably comfortable. When ministers as well as church leaders and congregations understand the consequences of Alzheimer's disease for both the sufferer and care givers, this is likely to be later rather than sooner. We must never overlook or underestimate the normalising power of genuine servant love. Caring, informed people can become keepers of the boundaries of independence and interdependence for those with diminishing life-skills.

To help local churches the following suggestions are offered:

- The congregation and leaders will be helped by an understanding of the nature and consequences of Alzheimer's disease in terms of behaviour, communication and life-skills. Information pamphlets are available from, among others, Christian Council on Ageing and MHA Care Group (formerly Methodist Homes). 'Understanding dementia', 'Visiting people with dementia' and 'Worship for people with dementia' are obtainable from MHA Care Group, Epworth House, Stuart St, Derby DE1 2EQ.

- The congregation and leaders should be aware of the implication of the demographic ageing trends for the Church and the community. In the UK and many other countries the number of elderly people is rapidly increasing. These are the ones God gives us now.

- Some knowledge of ways of communicating with older people with failing mental powers would be helpful and likely to ensure a greater sense of fulfilment in relationships. For instance, an understanding of the place of memory cueing can avoid embarrassment and added stress and confusion triggered by questions which seek information long lost. Here is a suggestion for a church door hostess to greet a person with Alzheimer's disease. (Notice that there are no questions.) Door Hostess:
'Good morning, Mrs J. Welcome to St Mark's Church. I'm Anne.

(Shakes hands, etc.) When my children were small you were the person who greeted me at church. This is your Order of Service/Prayer Book (handing items over). Mr P will see you to a pew.' (Indicates Mr P who walks with Mrs J to a convenient pew and places the hymn book in her hands with a smile.) All this would be said with natural pauses between sentences. It should be spoken clearly and deliberately, with a friendly tone and with few movements so that eye contact is maintained. If Mrs J is alone perhaps another person can sit with her ready to assist if needed.

- Congregations with a predominance of older people will need to give some thought to the availability of toilets which should be clearly signposted and close to the worship centre.

- The length of the worship service must also be taken into account – anything over the hour is likely to be stressful for older people and should be avoided.

Speaking at an Australian conference on ministry with seniors, Elbert Coles told of experiences of toilets when travelling with his seriously confused and memory-impaired wife. Something so simple as using a public toilet can become a nightmare for a care giver travelling with an Alzheimer's disease sufferer. Can she manage by herself? No, she can't. What to do if she goes in there on her own? Will she get upset and so confused that she comes out with her pants around her neck, on her head, or even left in the toilet? Or will she manage everything until she is confused by another way out of the toilet and becomes lost and frightened? And will she be ready when our flight is called? Should I go into the toilet with her and risk the screaming outrush of affronted women? These are not the dilemmas anyone would wish upon their worst enemy. Coles has attempted to solve the problem by championing the provision of 'family rooms' with toilets at airports and other places where the travelling public congregate. In these a mother of an intellectually disabled teenage son can supervise his toileting; a father can supervise his little girl needing to use the toilet and a spouse can give necessary help to a severely confused and memory-impaired person.

Such facilities are now appearing in airports and must be made available in places of worship so that people with early-stage dementia and their relatives can experience their customary worship as long as possible. It is becoming fashionable for churches to advertise themselves as 'inclusive' in their worship but even some of these have overlooked the reality that their physical facilities actually exclude many with early-stage brain and memory impairment.

The foregoing basic suggestions should help to empower elderly confused people to remain within the normal Sunday worship service, but in time they will not be enough. When that time comes no one should feel failure. As yet there is no way of defeating the consequences of Alzheimer's disease. Instead of lamenting this we should be rejoicing and giving thanks that, albeit imperfectly, our support has provided for as near normal quality of life as is possible for a time.

Worship in people's own homes

There are people who, although seriously disabled, can live at home because a family care giver, generally an elderly spouse or single daughter, is able to provide the necessary help.

Dr Anne Opie, senior research fellow with Health Services Centre, a joint venture between the Institute of Policy Studies, Victoria University of Wellington and the Wellington School of Medicine of the University of Otago, has edited an enlightening book of conversations with care givers of people with Alzheimer's disease and related disorders (Opie 1991). The book is particularly valuable and unusual in that she has allowed the reader the rare opportunity of reading a verbatim report of each interview.

Names are changed but the conversations are authentic. John Fuller, in his late seventies, cares alone for his wife Enid who has second-stage Alzheimer's disease. John tells Opie about their experience with their church:

> We haven't been to church for the last two years… We hardly ever missed before this. I noticed my wife was getting more and more uncertain about what to do at communion – whether to stand up, or kneel, or what – and she couldn't find her way to her seat. And I had to find all the hymns for her. Then, well, I got the feeling from one woman who used to engage Enid in intense conversations – I got the feeling it was with the purpose of seeing just what stupid things she'd say – quite possibly wrongly – but that upset me a lot. And then the minister left – so we haven't been since although I was involved with the church from the time I was a young man. I was an elder for nearly 50 years and held a lot of offices.

The complete verbatim account gives the strong impression that no one visited John Fuller to enquire about his absence from his church although it seems one couple did invite him to visit once or twice while Enid was in respite care. I do not know why the church forgot John and Enid. He may have been a difficult person. However, it is likely that John and Enid just dropped through the cracks in the pastoral care network. It happens all too frequently and no one individual feels a sense of responsibility.

Whenever I read the story of John and Enid I feel an immense sense of shame and sadness. I am part of the Church and cannot slough off incidents of pastoral indifference and ungraciousness. Certainly, overwork in the pastoral area is as dangerous and stressful as anywhere else and I am not denying the need for pastors to safeguard their own health and fitness. But too often we fail to set priorities in pastoral work and then cry 'overwork' when most of our week has been taken up in meetings and programmes which may feed our own egos and undermine our vocation. We must ensure that we attend to the needs of all those the Church has been given. Jesus said, 'those who lose their life for my sake, and for the sake of the gospel, will save it' (Mark 8:35). Quite clearly, there is nothing about wrapping ourselves in cotton wool to protect ourselves from the awkward needs of our neighbours. Only honest examination of self and God's grace will save us from too much carefulness.

Happily, there are more positive stories from some other parishes. They have involved small groups of six or seven people who have lovingly enabled a care giver to bring his or her spouse to worship almost to the time of death. These little support groups bestow an immeasurably precious gift. Alzheimer's disease exacts a long and arduous commitment, extending through perhaps eight to nine years or more.

Eventually, however, a time comes when it is no longer possible for most people with Alzheimer's disease to cope with the ordinary Sunday morning service. This needs to be acknowledged and some careful pastoral work should take place when the time is evident. A caring and informed pastor will be aware of the right moment to take the initiative. It is surely also necessary to take cognisance of a departure which is premature because of preventable causes. The Church has still to work through a theology which would guide its response to dementia. The Dementia Working Group of the Christian Council on Ageing is presently engaged in this task. However, changing attitudes is a daunting task.

Christians claim that the worth and sacredness of life rests in the graciousness of a God who loves and accepts no matter what the quality or condition of the one loved. The Church is meant to be the bearer of this grace. It is at its best when it provides adequately for all ages and conditions of people in its life and worship together.

When old people with brain failure can no longer cope with the local church's normal Sunday worship services, worship should be taken to them. If these people have been regular communicants a carefully shortened liturgy of holy communion is the most suitable form of worship to offer. A home communion or house mass is often deeply meaningful and thankfully received by people who respond to little else. I acknowledge that abbreviating the mass may be difficult for Roman Catholics but I am encouraged to believe that the essential elements of the liturgy can be retained without loss of integrity. The words of the key responses of the people are deeply embedded in the memory. The words, the chalice, the bread and wine, the actions and vestments of the president of the eucharist are powerful memory cues for those for whom the eucharist has always been a part of life and an essential spiritual resource. It is good to have a few family members or friends present to assist with the hymns and responses.

Lay ministers in some denominations can be trained and authorised to conduct the reserved sacrament from the church celebration to people's homes. A faith community which has a tradition of lay celebration of the sacraments in the absence of an ordained minister has a significant opportunity for pastoral ministry in the home setting. Lay ministers offering for this service should manifest a profound and sincere commitment to serve Christ in this way; their lives should demonstrate their fitness to exercise this ministry. A commissioning service will place this ministry in the context of the whole faith community, affirm gifts and strengthen the people involved. Great care should be taken to avoid giving the impression that the ordained minister is 'too busy' and so a 'second best' is arranged for shut-ins.

Care-givers will have their own beliefs and expectations and these must be talked through with the ordained person if necessary. Everything possible must be done to cue or trigger the disabled person's memory so that he or she may enter into the communion as fully as possible. Although we may feel inadequate in this ministry we can claim the presence and help of the Holy Spirit. I can think of very few commitments which warrant precedence over those for which the presbyter was specifically set aside in ordained ministry: word, sacrament and pastoral care.

Some people will not feel comfortable receiving communion often, others will have no sacramental tradition at all. For these a short service of word, prayer and praise may meet their needs. Both services will be more meaningful if the 'tools' I discussed in Chapter 3 are incorporated: orientation to the present reality, affirmation of feelings, memory cueing, and effective communication with confused, memory-impaired people.

Worship in a care home, hospital or day care centre

Worship is not an exclusively intellectual experience. We sometimes forget that people were worshipping God long before the majority could read or write. They certainly could not have understood long intellectual sermons. Jean Vanier, founder of the L'Arche communities, speaks of the rich and meaningful worship of severely intellectually impaired adults. Children are capable of worship without the developed intellect of most adults. So there is no valid excuse for neglecting to provide worship for people with dementia. Modern Western people value cognitive development and ability enormously, so it is small wonder that Alzheimer's disease, and other neurological disorders which drastically diminish reasoning powers, remembering and thinking, are so greatly feared. Human beings want to believe that the slippery nature of much of our living could be controlled if only we were able to *think* about it enough.

We think we can think God. The unknown author of *The Cloud of Unknowing* (Blackhouse 1985) had a different view:

> Your question once again draws me into that same darkness, that same cloud of unknowing in which I want you to be! For although we can, through grace, know and think about the workings of most matters and even those of God, yet of God himself no man can think. Consequently, I would set aside everything that can be thought about and choose for my love God – whom I cannot think about! Why? For the very fact that he can be loved and not reasoned. By love he may be sought and held, but not by thought.

Thinking and cognitive ability are important but not all that important in this thing that really matters: the true knowing and worship of God who 'by love may be caught and held but by thinking, never'.

The person with Alzheimer's disease may be incapable of ordered thinking, but we know, from the work of Brown and Ellor (1981), that the ability to feel remains intact. If we can cue the faith memory for a person with Alzheimer's disease we re-mind her or him of a former experience of God known in relationship. Along with worship this resurrection of experience and the feelings associated with it will be felt as part of the present moment. If the feelings are of love, thankfulness, adoration, joy and awe, that person, although sadly and undeniably limited, is participating in true worship which is acceptable to God. God is known in the experience.

Most people with Alzheimer's disease who have been worshipping church members in the past continue to recall some of the repetitive responses of the liturgy, prayers, hymns and psalms and patterns of worship that were memorised when they were young. If these memories go back to early childhood it is likely that not only will there be more of them but also that they will be stronger. (This is one vital reason for children continuing to be included as full participants in Sunday worship as well as memorising scripture, creeds, prayers and hymns. The big question is not worship or Christian education, but how can we best give our children an appetite for both?)

Liturgy, bread, wine, responsive prayer, cross or crucifix, candles, incense, stained-glass windows, prayer beads, music and even the vestments of the worship leader are all strong memory cues into worship. Those whose tradition includes some or all of them are more fortunate in forgetfulness and confusion than those of the 'plainer' Protestant traditions where variety and change in worship patterns, extempore prayer and strong emphasis on the sermon are the norm. In such traditions there is little opportunity for very much, except the hymns, the Lord's Prayer (older version), one or two psalms and a few verses of scripture to become deeply imprinted on the memory. The reader will notice that all these involve words, listening and thinking: the very abilities the person with brain failure is fast losing.

It is sometimes a good idea to invite the help of alert, mentally able people of a similar age and life experience to make a list of their favourite hymns and memorised scripture verses. The intention is that the list will encompass those hymns and scriptures, and even short prayers, which elderly confused people are likely to be able to be cued into. Another good idea is to try to take a look at Christian education materials which were used around the years 1920 to 1940 to find material which could be useful to cue people into a worship experience.

In my church tradition, sixty-plus years ago, little children sang, as the offering was received:

Hear the pennies dropping;
Listen while they fall.
Every one for Jesus;
He shall have them all.

Recently I used a suitable tape recording of this little song with a small group of elderly confused and memory-impaired Methodist men and women. One, who rarely communicates, stopped, stood up and stated firmly, 'I want to give something to Jesus. What can I give?' Someone else quietly said, 'A penny's not much' and was answered with, 'It isn't either. But God is good – we have enough – not much, but enough.' That moment was pure joy. I wonder if the person with dementia has a kind of wisdom from deep within his or her being? From what part does it come?

A friend attending a service of worship for seriously impaired people with dementia asked, 'Eileen, do they understand the scriptures we read for them? Do they understand that old prayer of confession?' My answer has to be, 'Probably not – not with their minds, anyway'. But the familiar language, helped by the symbols in the worship setting, can resonate through their bodies, re-minding them and re-membering them into the faith community. I think there is an affective kind of knowing. If we cue the faith memory in worship, love and a sense of presence are felt, and for a little time the personal identity is restored. Jesus has said, 'Where two or three are gathered in my name, I am there among them.' The Holy Spirit is a constant help, present and working.

However, the cueing of the memory does have its problems. Dora was born into a strongly evangelical Presbyterian family and until the age of 24 had seldom experienced any other worship tradition. Then she married Mike and converted to Roman Catholicism. She worshipped devoutly in that tradition for fifty years. Now, suffering the confusion and memory loss of Alzheimer's disease, she has no memory of those years. Now, it is her evangelical Presbyterian worship experience that cues her into worship. Try to imagine the shock of her parish priest when she sent him packing with 'We want none of your popery here!'. Imagine also, if you can, the confusion and sadness of her family and the loving generosity of the spirit of both priest and family as Dora continues to attend Protestant worship in her care home where I have the privilege of being her pastor. When Dora dies she will have a Roman Catholic funeral and I hope to be there.

Service of the word

I have found it best to organise worship around four basic elements. These are:

1.   favourite bible readings

2. well-known and well-loved hymns

3. patterned liturgical responses – most traditions have familiar statements of praise and prayer responses which are well embedded in the remote memory

4. prayer.

The tools – memory cueing, orientation to present reality, affirmation of all feelings and the principles of communication (discussed in the previous chapter) will all be useful to worship leaders who need to train themselves to apply them automatically wherever they are applicable.

Memory cueing

I always wear my clerical collar, ecumenical alb, stole and cross, and observe the colours of the liturgical year when leading worship for people with Alzheimer's disease. Some ministers feel they should not 'dress up' (their words) in the informal setting of the care home lounge. However, it needs to be understood that such memory cues are necessary to help many worshippers cue into 'church'. The care home lounge is now the only church space that the residents are likely to experience. I want to do every possible thing to make it a holy place of presence for them. That means clerical dress and vestments, flowers or candles, and a cross on the covered mobile feeding tray likely to be doing duty as an altar or communion table.

More than this is required, of course – a good deal of praying long before, a conscious claiming of the company of the Holy Spirit and a complete dependence on the work of the Holy Trinity to build community, harmony and order.

When lay people lead worship for people with Alzheimer's disease they should take care not to dress too informally. Wearing a clearly recognisable cross is very helpful. It would be helpful if there were some kind of agreed vestment for accredited lay preachers who do so much to bring God's word to old people in rest homes and hospitals. It would help elderly confused people if they had some distinguishing feature to aid a connection to the Church. For Methodists there is no reason why they should not be given the privilege of wearing John Wesley's preaching bands (without the clerical collar), and so that there could be no confusion they could be coloured rather than white. Deacons who take worship to people who are confused should wear the vestments appropriate in the Methodist or Anglican traditions. Worshippers are helped by these visual clues. The connotations of 'high' or 'Roman' – buried deep in some Protestant psyches – are irrelevant and have been for a very long time.

In one ward I visit for worship, as soon as one elderly confused gentleman sees me and my clerical collar, alb and stole he exclaims, 'Church!' and straightens his collar, tie and back. Another, at the beginning of a celebration of the eucharist, observing my collar, alb and stole, confided to his nurse sitting beside him, 'It's the priest. He's a lady.' Women clergy were not part of that man's remote memory. I had wondered if that would make it more difficult for the special people in my congregations. Apparently not.

Often I chuckle inwardly and wonder just what remote memory is being cued. One of my people, previously prominent in national public life and usually quietly composed and reverent during worship, was heard to exclaim during the short great thanksgiving prayer at the heart of the communion service, 'Dear God, I'd rather give a donation than sit through this!' Was he really cued into church or was it some public meeting? Anyway, how many of us have at some time longed to say the same thing half-way through a poorly prepared and delivered sermon on Sunday morning?

Familiar scripture is an effective memory cue. The call to worship, the assurance of forgiveness and the benediction are good places to use familiar scripture in worship. The content of worship material must be taken into account so as not to have a negative effect. Scripture passages ought not to stress sin and guilt, judgement and punishment. The overall message should be a positive one of hope, love, peace and God's abiding presence. I have found the following call to worship helpful for people with dementia. It orientates us all into the ultimate reality:

Minister: God is here.

People: God is always here.

Minister: God is with us.

People: God is always with us.

This positive note is important because many elderly confused people will take only a word or phrase from a hymn, reading or prayer and repeat it over and over. I believe it is more helpful for them to be reminded of God's love and mercy rather than God's judgement.

Some of the principles of orientation to present reality are used in the worship service itself. The tools of memory cueing, affirmation of feelings and relevant communication are also used throughout the pattern and content of the service. The call to worship is an example of all four tools being used effectively:

1. *memory cueing:* the worship leader's manner and dress
2. *reality orientation:* the statement, God is here
3. *feelings affirmation:* the statement affirms the sense of security the reality words convey
4. *communication:* eye contact, direct, simple, short sentence statement, announced clearly with confidence.

An order of service of word, prayer and praise

Greetings and orientation

Call to worship

Hymn

Prayer of confession

Assurance of forgiveness

Passing of Christ's peace (*visitors should be encouraged in this and what it demonstrates*)

Psalm or other encouraging scriptures

Hymn

Gospel reading

Good News sentences (*only two or three; short, simple concrete, relevant to the reading*)

Pastoral prayer

Lord's Prayer

Blessing

Benediction.

This service should take no longer than 25 minutes. Never shorten it by taking out the Call to Worship, a hymn or the Lord's Prayer; rather, take out a prayer and/or one reading.

The order 'works' for people at all stages of Alzheimer's disease and is completely suitable for a care home or hospital setting.

Leadership style

The worship leader needs to be confident and relaxed, and to speak in a clear, firm voice that can be heard by all. Instructions are best given in simple one-thought sentences, for example, 'We will pray', 'Hear God's word', and so on. For all worship, but especially for those in an advanced stage of the disease, I recommend inviting family and friends. This will not be possible in many care homes because their lounges were never designed for worship and are too small. Where there is a small church close by there are some compensations for the staff work involved in getting people there. Heating must, of course, be considered.

Care home management is increasingly realising the value of the spiritual dimension of care and these days is generally sympathetic. The climate of care is changing, and who knows? Nothing is lost by exploring a possibility. It is good to be able to lead the disabled in the responses and singing. Even if it is not feasible to invite family, it is usually possible to enlist the help of three or four people to come regularly to assist with responses and singing. In some care homes, after seeing the benefits of worship, staff members will sit with a patient to help and encourage them; this is a good bonding of helper and person being helped in the care home setting.

Practicalities of worship

The service should always be held on the same day of the week at the same time of day. The various elements of the worship should always appear in the same order. It is most desirable that the same worship leader take the service each week; if different people must be used they should be aware of the importance of using the same approach and the accustomed order of worship. Constancy assists with orientation. I would rather lead a weekly service for people with dementia at a care home and confine myself to three a week than lead 12 once a month at different homes.

It is useful to meet orientation needs by announcing the day, date and place and introducing key people.

> Good afternoon, everyone. My name is Eileen. I am the minister. This is Tom. He is playing the piano. We are at Sunnydale Nursing Home. You live here. Some of us are visiting you. Today is Tuesday 18th October. It is a beautiful autumn day. We have come together to worship God and to encourage each other.

I have found that hymn and prayer books are rarely used by elderly people in care homes. Even hymns in large print on separate sheets are hardly used. I have prepared large-print books with about ten of our favourite hymns but these are used mainly by visitors and, of course, are necessary just for that purpose. Many people with Alzheimer's disease like to hold a book or hymn sheet. One worship leader I know uses large-print hymn sheets in a plastic pocket and gives these out when necessary. Alternatively, they can be passed around to helpers (family or staff) sitting with the residents. Separate sheets are useful because they save people from the difficult task of finding the place in a hymn-book.

I do not use the overhead projector, despite its convenience. It is distracting in both noise and light and, more importantly, is not part of the remote memory of the people we serve. It is best to arrange everything so as to have as little movement as possible. Teachers of beginning readers run their fingers or pointers under the print, matching voice and word for their pupils, and this is a technique I have found useful and acceptable for elderly confused people. It works best when the helpers sit beside the residents. Sadly, that is not often due to lack of space.

I have found that hand gestures are helpful: the sign of the cross, the outspread half-circle arms of welcome and gathering in, and the raised arms for blessing. All enable communication. Participatory scripture is to be encouraged. This works well with the 23rd Psalm which many people in the age group we are considering have memorised in childhood. It will have to be in the Authorised (King James) Version, of course – avoid new translations and paraphrases which, you may think easier to understand, but we are not concerned so much with head knowing as heart knowing and for that the sound must be familiar. Hymns with a refrain such as 'Jesus wants me for a sunbeam' are also very popular.

For those situations devoid of music resources the Church's Ministry to Elderly Confused People has commissioned a most helpful audiotape, *Loving kindness in the land of forgetfulness* (available from Dementia Services Development Centre, University of Stirling). This has hymns grouped in threes, suitable for one service per set. There are hymns for Christmas, Easter and harvest festival as well as for ordinary days. Pitch and speed have been considered and suit the needs of elderly people. Old people can sing to the organ accompaniment and enjoy the tape immensely, not only during worship but also for quiet listening, especially in the late afternoon when some may be agitated and restless.

Since people with Alzheimer's disease tend to deteriorate in attention skills by the late afternoon it is best to plan worship for the late morning or early afternoon, say 10.45 a.m. or 1.30 p.m. Of course, it will have to fit in with the routines of the home.

Sometimes people in the earlier stages of the disease will be able, if invited, to request prayer for particular people or needs. I am always impressed and moved by their concern for others. The following are examples.

> We should pray for the church. The church is a big thing. I was a local preacher in the church. When the river flooded and the minister couldn't come then I took the service and preached. (Barbara)

> I want you to pray for the people who look after us here. (Andy)

> I get lost. Pray that God will always find me. It's awful to get lost. (Jane)

People in early-stage Alzheimer's disease will make a lot of comments seemingly unrelated to the worship service. As I am praying Bill will suddenly announce that he likes my hair or Claude will get stroppy and tell me that I can go to hell. Or dear little May will want the toilet urgently. It is all very testing and disconcerting at first and some worship leaders have absolutely no patience for it. I taught large classes of new-entrant five-year-olds for many years – the skill is in remaining quietly calm and confident and in using the seemingly irrelevant and occasionally irreverent interruptions in a positive manner to serve the worship. Some things, of course, are best just ignored.

Touch is very important to people with most types of dementia. Some years ago I was privileged to meet Mother Theresa of Calcutta. I have forgotten almost everything she said but I cannot forget the touch of her small, firm hand as she met my eyes and smiled. It is easier now to understand the great number of times we are told Jesus touched people. As I move about after worship I go to each person and clasp hands, meet their eyes with mine and sometimes hug people or stroke an arm or hand. I am aware of a special kind of meeting and my intuition tells me that the effects of all this touching at the close of our worship will remain with these people long after I have gone from that place. Indeed, the staff tell me that people are more relaxed and sometimes relate naturally to others. Once worship is established in a nursing home, staff notice the difference in residents who attend.

One morning I was standing in church when I became aware that we were singing a near-perfect formula for leading worship for people whose cognitive abilities are slowly and as certainly ebbing out like the ocean tide. It is worth sharing and remembering the essence of this simple hymn, which is to be found in many hymn collections:

Tell me the *old, old story*
of Jesus and his love.

Tell me the story *simply*
Tell me the story *slowly*
That I may take it in.

Tell me the story *often*
For I *forget* so soon.

Tell me the story *softly*
Tell me the story *always*
Tell me the *old, old story*
Christ Jesus makes thee whole.

Preparing worship for old people with failing mental powers often takes as long and as much effort and research as preparing the hour's worship of the normal Sunday service of any parish. Things that seem to be simple often turn out to be much more complicated than at first we thought. The foundation is prayer and the gracious work of God's Spirit. I may sometimes be discouraged but I am never dispirited.

For further information see Appendix 2.

The Lord's Supper

We must now consider that central rite in worship, variously known as the holy communion, the eucharist, the mass, the Lord's Supper. On the whole, in the context of a congregation of confused people, it is best to stay with a very much shortened and familiar liturgy. This is not a time for creativity – stay with the known. Take time. Name each person if possible: 'Mary, this is Christ's body, broken for you.' This helps to centre the communicant. Use small pieces of Lebanese bread (usually found among the pizzas in your supermarket) as ordinary bread will crumble when dipped in the wine and older people taking medication sometimes find wafers hard to dissolve. I always use unfermented grape juice rather than the usual communion wine; this is partly because of my own Church's tradition but also because alcohol and some medications may not mix well. Consult senior staff if necessary about what to use. Staff are helpful in providing information about a person's church denomination and commitment. We are not in the business of pushing religious rituals on to people who, if they could choose, would not want to receive communion. The relevant information may be available in the personal records but permission from family or an attorney may be necessary to gain access to these because of data protection regulations.

Sometimes with small groups of Nonconformist Christians I use the small individual communion glasses, but as care homes become larger and there are more residents of many different traditions to serve I mostly now use a chalice or common cup and dip the bread into the wine before placing it in the resident's mouth.

As in the home, I like to invite family members and friends to join the celebration. They are able to help with the responses and the singing, and a spouse, daughter or son will often respond positively to the invitation to serve their loved one. Visitors are invited to dip the bread for themselves. My experience is that these practices work very well with order, reverence and dignity, even if the procedure takes some time.

When serving the elements of bread and wine I find I have to centre my complete attention on the person in front of me as if he or she were the only person present. Often I find myself serving on my knees in order to make eye contact with residents sitting on chairs or in a bean bag on the floor. Although there will be a blessing at the end of the service I will bless each person as I move around the room. This touching and blessing is extremely important. In some care homes or hospitals where there may be fifty to sixty people to serve including residents and visitors it is very helpful to have two or even three people serving and someone playing the piano or a suitable tape of hymns. I have always been pleased when a Christian staff member serves the communion with me. At the Christmas eucharist we have invited children and babies; the older people love this.

Sometimes people hearing of our communion services will contest the whole thing on the grounds that the residents will not know what they are doing. Those who have witnessed and participated in these services would refute that. Very wonderful things happen. Sometimes people who have not taken one single initiative in many weeks – even months – will, when Christ's body in the bread is held before them, hold out their hands and say the Amen. Appreciation may not always be conventional. One day a most refined and well-spoken woman received the bread and wine very reverently and then burst out enthusiastically, 'Boy, that was good!' How true.

My first experience with holy communion and Alzheimer's disease was with my mother. I felt strongly that she needed the sacrament and would be comforted by it if she could be cued into it. I decided to take with me a very old book of bible stories. This was large and heavy, with a sober-looking cover. It had belonged to her when she was a child and she had frequently read the stories to me and my brother when we were small. It was a book of strong memories and associations for us all. I would use it with my mother before the sacramental liturgy. The old-fashioned black-and-white illustrations of our Lord on the Cross and the empty tomb of the resurrection morning awakened memories of our Lord's death and resurrection. This increased her confidence and enabled her to recall some of the responses and prayers. For a little time she felt her way into rich communion.

As I have taken the communion to more people, mostly in a large community setting rather than in their own homes or private rooms, I have come to appreciate that the gathering of the people in the presence of bread and wine provides most powerful cues to memory. How could it be otherwise? After the encounter on the Emmaus road: 'when he was at table with them, he took bread, blessed and broke it, and gave it to them. Then their eyes were opened and they recognised him.' (Luke 24:30–30). It still happens.

People are a little nervous when they first join us but soon that is forgotten. At first even I was concerned that some people might be offended if someone with dementia spat out the bread. I decided to wait and see. Anthony de Mello (1989) tells us a story I sometimes share with those who get anxious about what might happen in one of our celebrations.

He tells how a poor Italian family pleaded with their priest to be allowed to hold a wedding reception in the courtyard of the church. When it rained they asked for the further concession of moving into the church itself. Laced with alcohol the party became a lengthy and boisterous affair and the priest grew more and more anxious. When he tried to call a halt the family protested that Jesus himself had been happy to attend such a celebration at Cana in Galilee. The priest replied that, whilst that was true, they did not have the Blessed Sacrament there!

We so easily miss the one important thing. And in my experience no one has ever spat out the bread.

Much more upsetting is the practice whereby the priest or minister decides that a person is no longer a person and cannot understand what he or she is doing, and therefore should no longer be offered the sacrament. One faithful dementing Christian lady has had this experience. Staff are convinced that Patty still recognises the sacrament as she is passed by. Remember that Brown and Ellor (1981) have stated that feelings remain intact and appropriate in people with Alzheimer's disease. Imagine that old woman's feelings as she sees the precious bread of life and the wine of our salvation pass her by. Patty's behaviour has changed dramatically: she cries a lot, she yells out and disturbs others. At other times she just withdraws into herself for hours at a time. The wholeness of her health is further broken and her spirit is hungry. I believe the Holy Spirit ministers to Patty but I am offended by her Church's hardness of heart.

Towards understanding personhood

In the light of Patty's story I want now to share my understanding of person-hood. If Patty cannot receive Holy Communion because a representative of the Church has pronounced her a non-person, when did her personhood depart? Indeed, when and how did she acquire her personhood? Is identity the same thing as personhood? These are valid questions for care givers and others with responsibility for holistic care, especially when we are told that Alzheimer's disease and other dementia types are sometimes referred to as 'a loss of self'. Theologians may differ and I must respect their opinions even if I cannot, in the light of my life's experience, accept them.

One Sunday afternoon, a long time ago, a little girl aged about seven years, gumboots on her feet and best shoes clutched tightly one in each hand, ran across the home paddock and through the far paddock to the house of her great-aunts. They would take her to Sunday school where they were both teachers. They would go, as they did each week, not by car or bicycle or even Shanks's pony but by horse and gig. This was the only gig the little girl had ever seen, although her mother said there were a few old ones lying around untidy farmyards. The aunts' gig gleamed with 'elbow grease' (Grandfather said the aunts used a lot of that) but the child had never seen any in the harness shed although she had read the labels on every tin and jar which stood on the shelves.

I was that child. At Sunday school each child was given a card with a little picture and a short verse from the Bible. On the way home my task was to memorise that verse and reference. Once back at the house of my great-aunts I was rewarded for correct memorisation with a coloured boiled sweet from the big jar on the sideboard in their dining-room.

I have a very strong memory of difficulty with one verse. No wonder: it was 'Ye have received the spirit of adoption whereby we call Abba, Father' (Romans 8:15). Imagine that for a seven-year-old child – King James version and all. I could read it but I had no idea what it meant, nor did I understand the abbreviation for the letter to the Romans. However, I very much desired the waiting sweet so over and over I repeated the words. Eventually I got it right. As Aunt Ginny popped the lolly into my mouth she held my chin up and fixed my eyes with hers, saying gently but with all the authority of Sunday school teaching maiden great-aunts, 'It means, Eileen, that Jesus has made you a child of God'. A child of God! I am God's child? I am God's child!

All the way back across the paddocks I sang that miracle to the birds, the trees, the cows and the sky. 'I am God's child.' I accepted those words and I have never forgotten the verse. God's child! It is my deepest understanding of who I am and can never be taken from me. This is my true personhood – God-given, sacred. Nothing and no one can take it from me. It is the personhood too of those who, in their disease, can no longer remember. The very Spirit bears witness to our spirit that it is so (Gal 4:6). At the time of Holy Communion Christ is especially present to those who can no longer remember, making himself known in the breaking of the bread. These 'little ones' in mental chaos may be forgotten by others but God will never forget them.

Henri Nouwen (1998) explores ministry as 'remembrance' and the minister as a 'living reminder' of Jesus Christ. I simply am unable to believe that there could ever be a good enough reason for denying baptised people with Alzheimer's disease or other dementia the sacrament of the Lord's Supper. I would say to every presbyter: if you have no time for anything else in ministry to confused memory-impaired parishioners please take the sacrament of the eucharist regularly.

Understanding what is meant by identity

Whereas personhood is given to human beings by God, identity is given by others and the self. It is not always constant. We take our sense of identity from many sources. Identity can be lost or taken away or, sadly, forgotten. Parents give their children an identity as daughter or son. We have an identity according to the culture into which we were born and nurtured. A person's life work or profession may confer part or sometimes the whole of identity – which is why the 'empty nest' or retirement can be so stressful. Widows and widowers speak of feeling 'lost', of not knowing who they are, so closely has their identity been bound to another – the two become one.

Culture and our identity are extremely important. They are to be deeply respected. When memory is profoundly impaired human beings suffer a loss of identity and of self. They have been robbed of their sense of knowing who they are in relation to themselves, God (or the transcendent other), others and the environment. The remind-ing is a crucial pastoral task for ministers and care givers of people with dementia because 'knowing who I am' in relationship is central to spiritual health and well-being.

The opportunity to experience worship within the gathered community cues the remote memory, conferring again a sense of self in relationship to the creator God. Worship leaders can do a great deal to assist the older person with failing mental powers to experience worship. I see many who are, even for a little time, enlivened. I share the joy of a man who drives fifty miles each way to share worship with his old (and in other situations mostly unresponsive) Dad because, as he says, 'This is the one remaining thing that we can do together'. I observe the love in the eyes of a daughter as she serves communion to her mother and the surprised wonder of a new care giver in a large, noisy dementia ward when a reverent quietness descends as that lounge becomes a church.

It is a fact. 'God is here', initiating, restoring, calming and maintaining relationship with God's children. God is like the father who, seeing the lost son a long way off, hurried out to welcome him home.

Recently a fellow minister said to me:

> You know, John used to lead the worship in the dementia care nursing homes in the parish but now we've re-structured so that he can't do it. I'm doing it. I can't tell you how much I feared it or how much joy it gives me now that I've got over that. I see a small miracle every week. How many are given that?

People who live as helpers in Jean Vanier's L'Arche communities for severely intellectually and physically disabled people of all ages tell similar stories.

In this ministry I am learning to value my own memories. I find that the prayer which comes unsummoned to my heart just before I call our people to worship is this: 'Jesus, stand among us in your risen power.' Just so, my wonderful Sunday school teachers Great-Aunt Ginny and Great-Aunt Emma taught us to sing so long ago. And I wonder about the forgetful confused ones – are the memories cued for them in a similar way? Surely the community of saints is among us as unseen worshippers.

Examples of services that can be used with older people with dementia are to be found in Appendixes 3–6.

Summary

Many people with dementia are denied the opportunity for worship. Many more are denied the sacrament of Holy Communion. Gathering to worship in ways relevant to the special needs of people with Alzheimer's disease and other related conditions adds to their quality of life. Worship is a resource for spiritual health and well-being. The worship leader should plan worship so that memories are cued, feelings are affirmed and all communication takes into account the diminishing abilities of the congregation.

Worship services should be short and simple, but not childish. It is good to invite family and friends; they help to form community. The Eucharist or Holy Communion is the most suitable worship for those who have been regular communicants. Worship is always first and foremost God's initiative.

I have no way of actually measuring spiritual well-being and health or the extent of improvement to quality of life that results from worship and pastoral care which I describe in this chapter and the next. However, it is clear that some significant contact is made with many cognitively impaired people when they respond enthusiastically to familiar worship patterns and informed sensitive pastoral care. Certainly, the work being done with people with dementia contributes to the morale and the general health and well-being of care givers who often feel alone and unappreciated by the rest of society.

5

Being Present to the Person
with Dementia
The Pastoral Conversation

God told Moses: 'I'm in charge of mercy. I'm in charge of compassion.'
Compassion doesn't originate in our bleeding hearts or moral sweat but in
God's mercy. (Peterson 1993)

The friend who can be silent with us in a moment of despair and confusion
…who can tolerate not knowing, not curing, not healing and face with us
the reality of our powerlessness, that is the friend who cares. (Nouwen
1974)

In this chapter I describe a pastoral care approach which is relevant to the
special needs of older people with a dementia illness. This approach is
grounded in the belief that human beings are more than body, brain and
breath. There is a fourth dimension: spirit. The human spirit is capable of
reaching out beyond itself to the divine Spirit who calls the whole person to
eventual integration and wholeness.

There is a verse in the Book of Ecclesiastes which often comes to mind
when I am visiting a person with Alzheimer's disease: 'as you do not know
how the breath comes to the bones in the mother's womb, so you do not
know the work of God who makes everything' (Ecclesiastes 11:5).

So much happens in my pastoral encounters with older severely
memory-impaired and confused people than I ever expect or can possibly
explain. Much is mystery but there is also learning and insight.

This is a true story. I was principal of a city school. The small children in
the junior classes knew that my mother had lost her memory and were
always thinking of ways to help her find it. One afternoon two little boys
knocked on my office door and solemnly handed me two frogs in a jar.

'They're for your mother, to help her find her memory, Mrs Shamy,' they said.

Now the years have taught me that children often possess a wisdom long lost by adults so, crazy as it may seem, away I went after school to visit my mother, the two frogs in their jar with the gauze top on the passenger seat beside me.

As I walked into the lounge of the nursing home I was aware once more of this room of sad, silent, sitting women. It always seemed to me as if they had lost themselves and each other.

Each woman occupied her own silent reality while outside life pulsated urgently and noisily in the street, softly and busily murmuring in the early summer garden. But here, in this room, it seemed that life had quietly laid itself down, waiting for death.

I wanted to run back to life carrying the women with me. Instead I walked quickly to my mother's chair and, kneeling down in front of her, lifted the plastic gauze top from the jar. Instantly, in a quick green arc, one frog jumped on to her hand and then sat, very still. My mother pulled herself up straight in her chair and squealed with delight, 'It's a little frog!' And then, in quiet wonder, 'A little frog.' As her eyes met mine she softly said, 'I had a frog in a jar...'

As silently and as naturally as the light rises with the sun, banishing the darkness, so life entered that room, transforming the women, so that each one was sitting up straight, eyes bright and sparkling, darting here and there, following the frogs as they jumped in wide, quick leaps across the room and from one woman's lap to another. Soon the lounge was filled with a glorious pandemonium of delighted laughter, excited exclamations, joyous relationship and two tiny, quick, green frogs.

I watched spellbound as each woman was touched to life once more. This was resurrection. Everyone was talking at once in a happy determination to share the frogs. Then, amazingly, in a lull, I heard a woman singing:

> All things bright and beautiful,
> All creatures great and small;
> All things wise and wonderful,
> The Lord God made them all.

Can we explain what happened that day? My little lads at school were absolutely right. My mother had found her memory just as they hoped she would. Not only my mother but the other women, too, were re-mind-ed and re-member-ed into precious community. As I reflected upon this small miracle over the following days I was aware that most people of my mother's generation were the sons and daughters of pioneers who were farming the land. Each woman in that care home lounge had been raised in the countryside. In all probability each woman's childhood experience included frogs. Certainly our mother had sometimes shared with my brother and me her own childhood memories of looking for tadpoles and frogs in the farm pond and little creeks. She liked frogs, she knew about frogs and the frogs sent by the two small boys had acted as a powerful memory cue of other frogs in other jars long ago. With the return of that memory some of the joyful wonder-filled feelings of the original experiences filled her – and the other women too – and all of them were affirmed and validated by their sense of relationship and community and the gift of a common experience.

The memory of what happened in the care home lounge that afternoon was soon forgotten but we can conclude from the work of Brown and Ellor (1981) that the good, pleasant feelings would remain much longer. In fact, staff members were able to tell me that the women continued to relate in small ways for some time and were more relaxed and contented.

People are changed and brought nearer to wholeness as the human spirit is nourished and strengthened to reach beyond itself to a greater power, larger, loving and eternal, which wills even cognitively disabled people to sense meaning and purpose, bringing them to a balancing of integrity and despair which is the last developmental task of all human beings.

That there are blocks which hinder this final work for people with dementia is not denied. Their existence is cause for a spiritual dimension to their care. Most of us, however, do not start our relationship with people with Alzheimer's disease or any other kind of dementia illness so well. For most, their encounter with people with dementia in its latter stages is intensely disturbing. Una Knoll, a retired English doctor and deaconess, has written (*Ageing* 1990):

> I have a vivid memory of the fear and disgust that overwhelmed me when as a young medical student I visited a pscyho-geriatric ward full of senile old ladies. I was inexperienced and gauche, I did not begin to know how to talk to anyone. The patient who had been assigned to my care for the day called for her mother in a high-pitched whining voice at ten second intervals for the whole morning. It was a tremendous relief when she even-tually stopped whining while she gobbled up her lunch and then slumped

into her chair for her afternoon sleep. When she woke up she was wet, smelly and irritable. The whining started again, interspersed this time with a rich variety of swear words that embarrassed me. As we made our way to the bathroom door to change her clothes one of the older nurses said to her, 'You are a naughty girl, today, Rosa, playing up the young doctor like that.' Rosa stopped, swung herself around to face me, bared her gums in a ferocious grin and said in a clear voice, 'She doesn't like me and I don't like her so there!' It was true. At that moment I wanted to run away.

Although there is a growing public awareness and better understanding of dementia illnesses and of the people who suffer them (largely due to the work and commitment of the Alzheimer's Society) and, although attitudes and institutional caring modes are often more positive and caring, our society, including the faith community, still does a lot of running away from people with dementia. It is still not unusual to hear clergy and even family and friends covering their fear and embarrassment with statements like 'What's the use? She's off with the fairies', or 'He never remembers my name, let alone my visit', or 'I feel I just don't make any difference at all – there's never any change in him'. And quite commonly and frequently, 'I never see any progress or improvement for my time. Surely it's better to give my time where it counts.'

These comments exemplify our culture's high regard for doing, progress, usefulness and the profitable use of time. It is not easy to break with these values and relate to people in a different way.

At the beginning of my ministry to people with dementia I spent six months working in a pastoral capacity in a psycho-geriatric assessment ward as one of the requirements for my clinical pastoral education qualification. I remember very well my first day on the ward. Unlike Una Kroll and in spite of my experience with my mother, it was not so much fear and disgust I felt as an enormous and paralysing burden of helplessness, personal inadequacy and utter and absolute uselessness. It was a devastating experience and I, too, wanted to run away.

As a successful teacher and school principal with responsibility for a large staff, two hundred young children, the development of new curricula, a large budget and a complex of buildings, land and resources representing many thousands of dollars, I was accustomed – and indeed was expected – to control, objectify, categorise and facilitate. My expectations were for action and observable progress. Now none of that was relevant. I did not know how to be useful in my new environment. I felt like a five-year-old on her first day at school – miserable, inadequate and useless. I wanted to go home before someone pronounced that terrible word, 'useless', over me.

Alone that evening I pondered my sense of failure and shame, and I realised that part of it was being a New Zealander of pioneer stock. Very many New Zealanders are, at the most, only three to four generations removed from their pioneer settler forebears. A successful pioneer could turn his or her hand to almost any task and we are still, largely, a nation of handymen and handywomen. We make things. We fix things. We are task focused. We value doing. We value useful people and useful possessions. It has taken us a long time to value the 'useless' arts such as ballet and opera. By contrast, in Europe one will find many very ordinary people, not necessarily with tertiary education, enjoying classical opera and ballet. Not so in New Zealand – not yet. The very worst and most damning adjective my grandfather could use about a man, woman, child or beast was, 'useless'. In my culture it is a shameful thing to be useless. No wonder I felt badly. No wonder so many parish clergy are slow to offer pastoral care of a spiritual nature to people with dementia. The risk to self-confidence can be too great.

Before the harsh facts of an advanced dementia illness we are all likely to feel an enormous burden of fear and impotence. Fear, because in the company of Alzheimer's disease and other dementia disease we recognise ourselves as the future dwelling-place of old age, with all its losses and impotence, because we have learned to value doing above being and we do not know what to do.

'Useless' is the harsh verdict we pastors are in danger of pronouncing upon ourselves because we have been taught a mode of pastoral care (that is, a manner of caring for the whole person which is informed, gracious and intentional) which presupposes some intellectual abilities and capacity for insight in those to whom we are called. These are the very cognitive abilities which the person with dementia is progressively losing. The challenge therefore is to find a pastoral approach which takes cognisance of the need for an approach which is relevant to a person with a diminishing ability to think, to remember and to reason.

An appropriate pastoral mode

My attempts to find an appropriate model from an authoritative literary source failed. Seemingly, as recently as 1990 very little had been written about a successful pastoral mode for old people with failing mental powers. Although I spoke to some hospital chaplains, and found people working with intellectually handicapped people in an institutional environment, and discovered others who were ministering to people with mental illness in a hospital or community setting, and although all were understanding and encouraging, I had to conclude that if someone, somewhere had found a pastoral mode which was relevant to the needs of people with dementia and which included their spiritual needs, it would take time to find – and I was due back on the psycho-geriatric ward the next week. Added to that, I was fast becoming acutely aware of the needs of those people in the community whose dementia had been diagnosed and who continued to live in the community, either in a private dwelling (their own, or that of a family care giver) or in a private nursing home which cared for people in various stages of dementia illness. That led me to what felt at that time like a bold decision. I would allow people with dementia to teach me.

Back on the assessment ward I chose to see the residents not as sad, despairing and pitiful people but as wise people with their own wisdom and mostly happy people in their own reality. I decided to identify abilities (had I not been doing that all my working life?) and to stop lamenting deficits. I chose to relate in a different way. Instead of confronting ward residents with my reality I would try to be with them in theirs. I would try building person-to-person relationships and, remembering my little mother and following my own heart, I determined to enjoy my new friends. I gave up expectations as I chose to be with each one, attentive to each person's reality in the now of the present moment. I chose also to assume that at their age, like many others of similar age, they had completed the last task of Erikson's (1963) hierarchy of developmental tasks or somehow they were still, within their own reality, balancing despair and integrity. I have never felt completely useless again.

The pastoral care approach which developed, and which I still use with very few changes with people whose cognitive abilities are severely impaired by dementia illness, includes these four elements:

1.   mutuality – there is both a giving and receiving in the pastoral relationship

2.   a different way of thinking

3.   acceptance of the person

4.   a different way of relating.

These basic approaches to pastoral care with dementia sufferers are illustrated in this encounter with Kay.

Kay is in an early second stage of Alzheimer's disease – the confusional stage. Her memory is severely impaired, she has a very poor attention span now and the general decline of her intellectual abilities is readily discerned. She often cannot find the words she needs but is generally lively and enjoys being active with her husband in the garden and kitchen. Although her judgement is impaired her husband, Ken, is understanding and patient. They are both 76 years old. Kay is a retired nurse who worked part time after their children entered intermediate school and Ken is a retired company manager. I called early one evening and found it had been a hard day for Ken. They had received many visitors and, although they both loved that and Ken encouraged it, they were very tired and that had upset Kay so that she had become tearful and more confused than usual. Ken had prepared her for bed early and now hoped for a few hours of peace. After catching up with Ken I went up to the bedroom to see Kay in case she was still awake, which Ken thought was probable.

I went up the hall to Kay and found her sitting up in bed against her pretty pillows, lovely in her fresh blue nightgown, prim and proper, but with her pantyhose pulled down over her head, almost to her eyebrows. Whether by design or accident we'll never know, but the legs and feet of the pantyhose hung down each side of her head like long floppy ears. I stopped myself laughing – she looked so funny – and hugged her. She looked bewildered but smiled at me.

Eileen: I'm Eileen, Kay. Ken's in the kitchen. I've come to see you and – (*laughter bubbles out of me; I should not let it, I know, but as she moves her head the 'ears' swing – it is too much*). Oh, Kay, you've got your pantyhose on your head.

Kay did not think it funny. She drew herself up straight as a ramrod and, with all the dignified disapproval of a little Queen Victoria looked me up and down and said, slowly and sternly: 'And what would you do if you couldn't find your hairnet?'

Indeed, what would I do? Somehow I think I would not have been as creative as Kay, but then I do not live in Kay's reality of disorientation, confusion and forgetfulness. I realised that Kay was using a kind of wisdom to solve a problem from out of her reality. Her illness, her very forgetfulness, had directed her towards resolving her problem.

I have witnessed similar exercising of wisdom in face of the problems which dementia illness presents to those who must live in its harsh reality. I remember also my mother's wisdom: 'God never forgets us. Remember that, dear.'

Barbara Hanson (1989) supports my intuitive understanding that in my work with confused mentally disabled older people I am privileged to meet people often as figures of wisdom. Naomi Feil (1993) also asserts that her mode of validating the feelings of persons who are old and disoriented means that their wisdom is acknowledged.

Attitude, the way the pastor or carer chooses to regard the person with a dementia illness, is crucial to caring. The way society, the Church, the family and the institution – be it hospital or care home – looks upon cognitively impaired old people is a choice. Justice and compassion seem to suggest that we should choose to interpret their condition as one of integrity rather than of despair. I have learned to look on the people I work with as teachers with wisdom to share as well as persons needing special care. That is the core of my advocacy for them.

The basics

The four basic elements which ideally should be present in any pastoral/caring encounter with the person with a primary dementia illness can be identified in the verbatim conversation recounted above.

Mutuality

Kay claimed mutuality when she rebuked me. I should not have laughed. While we remained in our own personal reality I viewed her as lacking reason and she obviously didn't appreciate my evaluation of her which my laughter revealed. Only when I endeavoured to enter her reality with a small measure of success could we begin to relate. The pastor or carer giver must make that move because Kay and those like her cannot.

A different way of thinking

The conversation illustrates powerfully the kind of thinking which can shape our normal everyday attitudes and judgements. Only by an endeavour to view Kay's situation and behaviour from a reality which is not my own but Kay's am I brought to an understanding of the difference that makes to my evaluation of her abilities and behaviour. Although she looked foolish she had actually been very resourceful.

Pastors and care givers must use that kind of perception to understand how it might alter their view of what is reasonable and logical. We may well discover that within his or her own reality the person with dementia possesses a certain wisdom. It was so with Kay.

An acceptance of the person

I attempted to offer, in spite of the humour of the situation, an acceptance which was complete and unconditional. This quality of acceptance is healing for those whose disease cannot be cured.

A different way of relating

It was necessary for me to adopt a style of relating which respected Kay's personhood. The visitor must show acceptance which is responsible but does not seek to be controlling. If the pastor can 'connect' with the person whose reality is not the same as his or her own, that will increase the power of the dementing person. This is certainly not easy at first. The more experience of relating to many people with dementia the pastor and care giver have, the easier it will become.

Mimesis is one technique which can help the pastor and care giver enter the world of the person affected by a dementia illness and identify with him. It involves imitating the person's behaviour and copying his affective – or feelings – range. It is not a comfortable technique because it involves skill in copying a person's mannerisms such as the way she holds her cup or the way he walks and sits, and so on. It is probably more successful practised on a regular and frequent basis. It also includes learning to play and have fun. This is play as children play. In my world and the world of a care giver or pastor such play is called pretending. For the person with dementia it is the reality of the now. I quite often take 'tea' with one of my people. Rather than confronting a person with my reality which means cups, a teapot or at least tea bags, hot water and so on, I enter her reality which finds none of these necessary. This does not mean I relate to a person with dementia as if she were a child. All that is done must honour and respect personhood.

These four elements of a successful pastoral mode for people in the circumstance of dementia are factors controlled by the pastor or care giver's attitudes.

Other factors influencing spiritual health and well-being

Other essential factors which shape spiritual health include:

- a sense of identity
- a sense of relationship with God, self, others and with the environment
- a strong sense that life has meaning and purpose.

A sense of identity

The identity of each person is defined by who that person is in relationship to self, to other people and to the environment. The self, other people and the environment may bestow a person's identity. Personhood, as we have already noted, is different; it is defined by relationship to God. Personhood cannot be taken from us because it is God-given. When others attempt to deprive a person of his or her personhood we call it oppression. Personhood is our essential dignity as human beings made, Christians and Jews believe, in the image of God. For Christians personhood is defined as 'child of God'.

Because we know that the person with Alzheimer's disease or other primary dementia-type illness will gradually lose the sense of his or her identity, the task of the pastor will be always to remind that person of who he or she is and when that is no longer possible to see that his or her identity is preserved by the person's community. It is the solemn obligation of the Church, the body of Christ, to remember for those of the faith family who can no longer themselves remember.

The foundation of my understanding of who I am as pastor or care giver to a person with advanced dementia is not what I see before me but what God in Christ has said and done. No matter what the condition of any human being, his or her personhood in God requires that pastor and care giver come before that person in reverence. Family, friends, care givers and the faith community can all help maintain a sense of identity for the person with Alzheimer's disease. At one of my seminars I met a young male care giver who confessed that he had always felt very negative and irritated beyond words by a certain very old man who was slow and shuffling and so confused that he had forgotten his identity. Once the young care giver learned that the man was a former All Black he found a new respect for his patient and loved talking rugby with him, reminding him of his former identity.

A sense of relationship

Human beings are only truly and fully human as they are in relationship with others. One of the tasks of the pastor and care giver is to promote sociability among people with dementia. One of the very important things that happened when I took the frogs to my mother's nursing home lounge was that the common experience and the raised memories brought those silent, isolated women into relationship with each other.

One of my warmest memories is of visiting a day care centre for people with Alzheimer's disease in Scotland. The staff person introduced me to a room of silent men and women, totally lost within themselves. There was absolutely no response until I asked to be introduced personally to each person. I was taken to a seemingly lost and unaware old lady. 'Eileen, this is Ethel.' And quite spontaneously I exclaimed, 'Oh, Ethel. Ethel is the name of my mother-in-law.' What a transformation. Suddenly Ethel was sitting up straight, eyes bright and with a smile that I am sure started in her toes, for I saw it encompass her whole body until it reached her face and she stretched out her arms to embrace me, saying 'Oh, my dear, we're related! We're related!' Then, with her eyes she gathered everyone in that room into our meeting, calling to them, 'We're related. We're related.' We were away – 'related'. Related in our common humanity, related in our singing and our talking – all together – and, wonder of wonders, in our dancing!

Of course it does not always happen like this. But when it does not happen a good pastor or care giver finds a way to initiate experiences of community relating. Ways will be found also for relating to the environment, especially the world outside the care home lounge. Opportunities for relating to God will also be present and not only in worship and prayer and hymn singing but also as the One who is revealed in all creation.

A sense of meaning and purpose

What is the meaning and purpose of life when a person is old and mental powers are failing to the extent they do in people with dementia? I continue to ponder that question and long for companions to ponder it with me. All that I am able to do from my own experience is to offer some reflection and perhaps push out the boundaries of the reader's frame of reference. Certainly the question demands more than a bio-medical paradigm.

One of our difficulties, I have come to understand, even in normal ageing, is the absence of symbols for transcendence and appropriate rituals to mark and give positive significance and meaning to the passing of life –

and I mean the whole of life – especially those stepping-stones which lead into older life, loss and dependency. Without these positive symbols and rituals to give meaning to growing older (which is what every alive person is doing and which our culture and churches mark reasonably well from infancy to adolescence) it is little wonder so much energy is devoted to staying young and the glorification of all things youthful, and to an irrational denigration and denial of the natural process of life, ending in death.

The Christian Church and other world faiths practised in the use of symbol and ritual to give meaning to the seemingly inexplicable surely have gifts to offer in this matter. Meaning formation in the last half of life is not a fringe benefit, an option to be offered by a few people sensitive to the needs and the demographic ageing trends of our time, but a major ministry.

According to Frankl (1978), if this work of compassion and common sense is not done, a kind of neurosis may develop. He calls this a 'noogenic neurosis', meaning that its origin is a spiritual matter. Could it be that a neglect of the spiritual dimension of care contributes in part to the total confusion of the person with dementia? That seems to be entirely possible. We know, of course, that confusion and impaired memory and other difficulties affecting behaviours and abilities in dementia are caused by changes in the brain structure. However, the work of Dr Tom Kitwood and others indicates that this confusion may be exacerbated by a mode of care which is excessively controlling and fails to respect individual differences (Kitwood and Bredin 1992). There is evidence to support the view that 'person-to-person' care not only enhances quality of life but may also slow down the extent and progress of confusion and memory impairment in people with dementia. By no means should we dismiss the spiritual dimension of care (or lack of it) as irrelevant to an increase of confusion not attributable to changes in brain structure.

In terms of spiritual neglect and confusion, one of our difficulties is our inability to measure spiritual health and well-being. What is needed is a paradigm which recognises the spiritual dimension for the comprehension and integration of human phenomena which is incomprehensible in biology and psychology. That takes us back to Catherine Benland's (1998) claim that we are more than body, brain and breath, even if that something cannot be measured. Is there someone somewhere who can translate the very real wisdom of the heart into language that is acceptable and understood by scientists?

Victor Frankl (1978) has written that life can be made meaningful in a threefold way, and I have found that it is possible to provide these three means for people with dementia.

1. GIVING TO THE WORLD

The first is by giving the person opportunities to give to the world: fulfilling or realising creative values. Care home management that allows residents to garden, wash and dry dishes and do other small tasks, as well as encouraging its residents in their hobby skills, such as knitting, are assisting them to do the spiritual work of giving their lives meaning and purpose.

In an earlier chapter I have related what happened to my mother when she lost her crochet hook and therefore was deprived of opportunity to experience her creativity and give to others the work of her hands. There was no provision for helping with such things as setting tables (as I have seen in some other nursing homes more recently), and since residents were forbidden in the kitchen she was unable even to dry dishes which she could have managed and really loved to do for me whenever I brought her home. It is unlikely that those who make such rules understand that spiritual well-being is denied when this happens.

Some of my readers may find this difficult to accept. It will help to recall a time in your life when, under a great deal of pressure, you were engaged in the same mental activity (or non-activity) for every waking minute. Perhaps you were swotting for important exams. Perhaps you were convalescing, unable to engage in any activity. Did you, towards the end of that time, yearn to do something creative with your hands like baking a cake, preparing and planting a garden plot, putting up a shelf or perhaps painting the shed? If you have had that experience you will know how poorly the human spirit becomes when deprived of opportunity to achieve a creative work, no matter how small or seemingly unimportant.

The Christian Church makes a significant contribution to people's spiritual health when it hosts such activities as craft clubs.

2. TAKING FROM THE WORLD

The second means for making sense of life and giving it meaning and purpose is that of realising or fulfilling experiential values. This means that the human spirit is nourished by experiences of love, truth, beauty and whatever is good and noble. Wherever these are experienced the human spirit is uplifted. Think of what a Beethoven sonata does for our drooping spirits.

3. REALISING OR FULFILLING ATTITUDINAL VALUES – A 'STANDING PLACE'

This means making sense of and accepting without despair and disintegration whatever circumstances life may throw up, even that most noble of values which is the acceptance of undeserved suffering without bitterness and death-tolling despair. This almost always implies the seeking of a faith system and the practice of the beliefs and rituals of religion. For Christians this means Christ Jesus, prayer, the sacraments, worship and discipleship, hymn singing, the study of the Bible and much more.

One of the pastoral tasks of the Christian pastor is to be an effective advocate of the spiritual dimension of care and to make effective representation to care home and hospital management wherever access to religious practice and rituals is denied.

Tools for the pastoral encounter

These are some tools that I use for the pastoral conversation or encounter.

An initial orientation to the present reality

Without confrontation, but gently and naturally, I try to orientate the person to the reality of the here and now in the simple everyday facts which impinge upon all. I do not expect to be remembered from previous visits, so I introduce myself on each occasion and I always wear my clerical collar which almost always gives a severely memory-impaired person a visual cue to recognition of my function and identity. I might also introduce the name of the day and perhaps the season or weather or other snippet of information topical to the day and person.

I really do not know how helpful this is to the person with dementia but sometimes I am surprised by the connections made and this happens often enough for me to believe it to be worthwhile.

If I can help restore identity even momentarily to a person who only fleetingly and partially knows him- or herself, that is not a waste of time. During 1992 I visited a Methodist care home in Nottingham where a fine intentional programme integrating the elderly physically frail and the elderly mentally frail was practised. When I was talking to a resident suffering some kind of dementia illness I introduced myself as a clergywoman, telling her my name and that I came from Christchurch in New Zealand. She responded with the information that she had visited Christchurch twice. The staff person with me thought that this response came out of her confusion but I was not so certain; her eyes had brightened and she had nodded and smiled when I spoke of Cathedral Square, the Avon River, Cashmere Hills and daffodils in Hagley Park. Although she actually said nothing beyond that initial response, 'I have been to Christchurch twice,' I was sufficiently intrigued and connected to seek out her frail but cognitively able sister who also lived in that nursing home. Sure enough, she told me that her sister had indeed visited my home city twice, once as an exchange teacher for a year and once as a visitor on holiday.

The sense of relationship with this lady was strong enough for me to remember her long after our meeting. Did she feel it too? Was the orientation worthwhile? We cannot know for certain; however, I believe that somewhere from an 'island of knowing' in her brain came recognition of the words 'Christchurch, New Zealand' sufficiently sure for us to be connected in a common experience. For a brief moment we were in a meaningful relationship and she knew herself as someone who had visited that faraway place.

The affirmation of feelings

During the pastoral visit I am aware that I am listening, paying attention on two levels: on one I am hearing a lot of confusion and on another (deep in my gut) I am paying attention to the feelings behind the words. These, I believe, reveal that reality experienced at that time by the person with me.

Robert Davis (1989), writing about his own experience of Alzheimer's disease, relates that his worst personal loss was the spiritual change he noticed. He felt fear. He writes that he feels like 'an orphaned child, lost, abandoned and never found'. From out of his personal experience of early-stage Alzheimer's disease he is able to write of what helps him in that fear, and it is definitely not reasoning and logic. He asks instead for the comfort of the reassurance that he will not be abandoned and he asks for a gentle voice with calming words or songs accompanied by appropriate and consoling touching. In other words he is asking that his feelings be affirmed (pp.123–124).

Very often when I first enter a care home I will be met by a staff person requesting me to go to an old man or woman 'who has been crying all morning'. Why is this old person crying? Perhaps I see an old man, 86 years old, sobbing like a small child. He is crying for his mother. This old man wants his mother. He is 86 years old and his mother has been dead many years; how can she come? This is confusion. In my reality what he asks for is crazy, unreal. But I am paying attention at another level (the Carmelite Sisters suggested to me that this is prayer) to the feelings this old man expresses in wanting his mother to come to him.

What are we feeling when we cry for our mothers? Could it be fear? That fear of aloneness and lostness of which Robert Davis writes? I believe that is entirely possible and my heart goes out to an old man as if he were a small frightened child and I comfort him as I used to comfort my small sons. I put my arms around him, making the small comforting sounds all mothers know and I tell him it is terrible to be afraid and alone, that it is very, very hard to be left alone. I tell him I care, that I will stay with him until he is feeling better. After a little time he is able to stop crying and if he is mobile I will take his hand and we may walk together. When it is time to go I do not leave him sitting alone and isolated but I give him something to hold, a large soft toy or perhaps a holding cross. If he is a Christian we might pray the Lord's Prayer or say the 23rd Psalm together. I make sure he is sitting with others and I tell him the names of the people next to him and, as I leave, I take his hands in mine, make eye contact and assure him that although I am going now I shall be back. And I keep that promise. If it is appropriate I may ask a blessing for him.

My reader might ask, what of tomorrow? Will it be the same? It could be. The person with severe memory loss has no concept of the future. I shall not use precious energy pursuing that. What he does have is his reality of the 'now' in this present moment, and the feeling, now, of being cared for, of security and love which will remain much longer than a moment.

If I explain what I have done and why to his care giver, he or she may be able to do likewise and bring him out of his fear when he next enters it. This is likely to be the shape of pastoral care in this kind of situation. I find that once pastors realise that there is a healing work to be done and a way to do it they lose their fear and sense of inadequacy. They begin to see not a disease but a person and that makes all the difference. Care givers too, both family and professional, are empowered knowing this shape of caring which reaches the person with Alzheimer's disease.

I have tried to explain what I mean by affirming all feeling and by relating in a different way. I cannot emphasise too strongly the need to pay attention, to be truly present to the person in order to discern the person's emotional state and own personal reality. Regarding the case I have just related it may be helpful for readers to ask these questions of themselves:

- What did the pastor see?
- What did the pastor hear?
- Which is likely to indicate the old man's personal reality?
- What is the old man's reality?
- Is it the same as the pastor's?
- Whose reality does the pastor work in to provide authentic pastoral care?

Remember that feelings remain intact and appropriate well into the progress of Alzheimer's disease. The mode I have described above may not be so successful with other diseases or conditions causing dementia.

Of course such a pastoral encounter may not always be as easy. I illustrate with Jack's case. Only after the following encounter did any of Jack's nursing home care givers know that he had stayed a single man on the dairy farm with his widowed mother. If Jack was for some reason sick (and he had suffered numerous health problems) it was the old lady who had to do the milking. Seated beside a cow and later with machines, she had never forgotten the skill of milking cows. She had, however, become forgetful and confused in other ways and Jack had cared for her throughout this difficult time. This information had not been recorded on Jack's own records; although 'previous occupation' was shown as 'dairy farmer' it was not complete enough and the details were not known by the pastor or care giver staff. This makes the obvious although helpful point that it is useless recording information unless it is accessible to those who work with the person concerned.

Now physically frail and assessed as suffering Alzheimer's disease, early second stage, Jack lived in this beautifully presented and furnished care home. Nothing in this city home could possibly or even remotely cue his memory of his previous home. He has difficulty talking and usually says little more than 'Thank you' when helped or receiving.

However, most afternoons, soon after 4 p.m., he starts to indicate a restlessness and frustration. He is very frail and lacks the strength to haul himself out of his chair and is frustrated at every attempt. He reaches out to catch hold of anyone passing and begins a litany, 'Mum, are the cows in?' Most people are mystified and do not answer him, which only frustrates him further so that he strains horribly to get up from his chair and mutters anxiously about the cows.

It is very distressing for everyone but no one seems to understand the reason for his difficulty or how to help him. Gradually his voice becomes louder: '*Mum*! Are the cows in?' On and on it goes, getting louder and louder. Jack is beside himself with frustrated anger and anxiety. Someone on the staff demands that he stop but he is far too upset now to be persuaded to be quiet.

The new pastor comes in and looks over the whole lounge, noting that staff are very rushed getting people ready to go back to bed or setting up feeding trays for the early tea of rest homes. Seeing the pastor standing there seemingly doing nothing the staff nurse suggests he go to Jack.

'Jack? Oh, the one making all the noise.'

Imagine you are this pastor. You walk over to his chair and sit down. Jack grabs you. 'Mum, are the cows in?' What on earth – ? In this hospital, located on a busy city street? Cows? His confusion will probably confuse you; how are you going to 'reach' this man, you ask yourself. Your encounter may go something like this:

Jack:	(*grabbing the pastor's arm and holding on tightly*) Mum, are the cows in?
Pastor:	(*puzzled*) I don't know. Cows?
Jack:	(*shouting*) Mum, are the cows in?
Pastor:	(*feeling very uncomfortable now and wanting to break free*) I don't know... Cows?
Jack:	(*shouting even louder and gripping the pastor's sleeve. Other patients are now visibly upset*) *Mum*! Are the cows in?
Pastor:	(*desperate*) I don't know – I'll find out! (*He moves to the corridor feeling foolish and embarrassed. What to do now? He wants to duck off out to his car but Jack is still shouting and by the sound of him, almost beside himself with frustrated anxiety. In an inspired flash the pastor realises how it must feel for Jack. Now he enters Jack's reality and the feeling of foolishness is replaced by an enormous compassion. Back into the ward he strides and when Jack grabs his sleeve and shouts his frustrated question once more...*)
Jack:	Mum! Are the cows in?
Pastor:	(*With a huge intake of breath!*) Yes! The cows are all in. Don't worry now. The cows are in.

Jack: Oh, thank you. (*He relaxes, settles back into chair and closes his eyes.*)

Pastor: It's important to get them in on time.

Jack: (*still with eyes closed*) Yes, thank you.

Pastor: I'm glad the cows are in. (*He puts his hand out to touch Jack's shoulder. It is a strong and caring gesture, unselfconscious and spontaneous.*)

Jack: (*opening his eyes*) Thank you. (*He and the pastor make eye contact and smile.*)

Pastor: Thank you. And God bless you. I'll call again.

         (*Jack's eyes follow him and the pastor catches up with the staff nurse. She nods and he grins, pleased with the whole experience*).

The pastor reflected. What had really happened? When did the encounter begin to feel easy? Why? What did entering Jack's reality do for Jack? Did it affirm his feelings? Yes. What did entering Jack's reality do for the pastor? What did the pastor learn? This is a simple but positive pastoral encounter. Let us check it against our criteria.

- Was there mutuality? Yes, but not at first.
- Was there a different kind of relating and thinking? Yes, although it took time. That's OK – it does take time and insight.
- Was there respect and relationship? Yes.
- Was there complete and unconditional acceptance?
- Were feelings affirmed and reality for the person with dementia recognised?

Another question we might ask is, what tools did the pastor use?

Memory cueing

I discussed and described this too in Chapter 3. The function of memory is essential for the successful completion of the task of late life which, in Erikson's (1963) hierarchy of developmental stages is the forming of a sense of integrity (an understanding, a satisfactory insight and acceptance of why and how we have each lived our lives). In the latter life stage this is a work going on within us. It is not accomplished in an afternoon but is rather a process of review, reminiscence, remembrance and the recalling of the memories of our earlier days.

We have noted that, when the memory of a particular occasion comes to our consciousness, with it comes also some of the feelings associated with the original experience. That is significant for our caring and pastoral ministries because we know that people with Alzheimer's-type dementia have the ability to feel appropriately and to respond to feelings. If we can cue the remote memory we are providing an opportunity for the person with Alzheimer's disease to:

- recall a specific episode from the past
- have the feelings of the past experience in the present, recognised and affirmed
- communicate in the present by way of the past, thus allowing for relating to family and others. Reconciliation may be possible
- sense, even briefly, his or her own identity.

An example of the latter is when the frogs cued my mother's remote memory and she knew herself again as a woman who knew about frogs and enjoyed them. Because the other women seemingly had the same experience of some identity realisation it was possible for them all to experience relationship as a community. Although this relating was brief and probably quickly lost to them, the feelings remained long after. We know that a sense of identity and relationship are essential to spiritual health and well-being. If the pastor or care giver can cue the memory of the person with Alzheimer's disease she or he makes a significant contribution to enhanced quality of life for the sufferer. It is my experience that reminiscence, enabled by memory cueing, promotes socialisation. Without it, memory-impaired, confused elderly people living in institutions are rarely engaged in conversation. It is possible that the attendant absence of sensory stimulation hastens the decline of their cognitive and social abilities.

Charlotte, whom we met earlier, is an 80-year-old woman who has never married. She is a practising Christian although she has been unable to attend her church for some time. Charlotte graduated from university with an MA (Hons) in English literature. She is a retired schoolteacher, a nationally recognised artist and has held many responsible offices in voluntary organisations. She now lives in 'The Elms' nursing home after assessment and the diagnosis of Alzheimer's disease. She is very confused and socially isolated. When I first visited her, following a request from her sister, she was very withdrawn and kept herself apart from the other residents. She had 'run away' twice from her first placement but seemed to have lost a lot of her healthy awkwardness. I usually found her sitting alone on the terrace, waiting for someone to 'take me away from here. It is not congenial'.

On this visit, however, I found her in the lounge where an activities organiser was conducting some large soft ball exercises with the residents. I observed this until noticed by the organiser. I asked to see Charlotte who, I observed, was looking very glum and disapproving and having nothing – definitely nothing – to do with any large ball or resident.

Eileen: Hello, everyone. Excuse me interrupting. I've come to visit Charlotte.

Charlotte: (*hearing her name, she perks up*) Oh, a visitor. How kind of you to call. (*We move towards each other and Charlotte has her arm graciously extended ready to shake hands.*) Oh, yes, you were at that delightful meeting at Brighton. I remember your face so well. Such a happy meeting. (*This is pure fantasy – confusion – and I think also a little showing off and taking charge. Good for her!*)

Eileen: Good morning, Charlotte. It's good to see you so well. Thank you for making me so welcome. I'm Eileen. I'm the Methodist minister. I often visit you. (*Since there is no room to sit down beside her I drop to my knees on the floor by her chair.*) I visit you most Tuesdays. Today is Tuesday.

Nancy: (*Another resident who has been sitting in the chair next to the one Charlotte has now returned to with me in tow.*) Oh, please don't sit on the floor. Have you come to see me?

Charlotte: (*sharply*) Indeed not. We will go to my room. (*Said with a haughty shrug of her shoulders and raised eyebrows as she turns to me again.*) Well! Manners! Come, follow me... Oh, that meeting... On and on. They get nowhere, you know. (*We reach her room. There is one chair on which there is a pile of neatly folded dresses.*) This is it, my dear. It's only temporary. I'm moving out soon you know. (*Charlotte will not have her clothes in the wardrobe. She is always ready to move out.*) Now you'll have to sit on the bed. It's not what we're used to, but...

Eileen: That's fine, Charlotte. We'll move the clothes so you can use the chair.

Charlotte: This chair. Oh this chair. It's older than me. My legs are better, though. I first saw this chair when I was six years old. It is my grandmother's. See, it's loose here. I've tied it. (*She shows me.*) Now look at this cushion: I made that... (*She falters, seemingly lost.*) Well, I think I made it… I must have made it… (*She looks bewildered and vulnerable but quickly recovers.*) Well, it doesn't matter. It is these dresses I want you to see. I made them all. (*Grandly*) Yes, I made them all. (*She shows me the dresses, telling me her favourites, the sewing inadequacies of her sister, the price of the materials, and so on, non-stop*).

Eileen: You enjoyed dressmaking when you were younger, Charlotte?

Charlotte: (*Affronted*) Dressmaking? I was never a dressmaker. I am a teacher.

Eileen: (*This is reality and I try to go with it.*) Yes. You were a teacher. You were a fine teacher, Charlotte. English literature was your special subject. You recited Shakespeare for me when I was here to visit you last week. You recited Portia's mercy speech from *The Merchant of Venice*. You gave me so much pleasure, Charlotte. 'The quality of mercy…'

Charlotte: (*Excited and coming in quickly*) '…is not strained. It droppeth as the gentle rain from Heaven on the place beneath… (*She recites word perfect through to*) … the fear of kings.' (*Eyes shine, her body leans forward. Once or twice she falters and I prompt and join in for a few words. She nods and claps me.*) Oh, you are so good. You have improved. It is beautiful language. What an understanding of God. And such words. (*She is sparkling with pleasure, full of energy. Then she sits still as if listening. She closes her eyes. I wait in the silence. After a few minutes she begins to recite again, softly and hesitantly at first the opening lines of Milton's sonnet 'On his Blindness'.*)

Charlotte: 'When I consider how my life is spent,
                  'Ere half my life in this dark world and wide…'
                  (*She softly recites almost all of Milton's sonnet. Once, when she stops, I could prompt her, but twice she pauses and repeats the line until the next comes. Her memory of Milton is better than mine. When she had finished she sits composed and, it seems to me, filled with pleasure.*)

Charlotte: It's the most beautiful language in the world… You love it too?

Eileen: Yes, I do, Charlotte, I am very moved. What a treat you've given me. You're wonderful to remember Milton – not an easy poet.

Charlotte: (*Softly*) I love poetry. It is the music of my soul. (*We sit quietly, comfortable together in the silence. Then quite suddenly Charlotte straightens and stiffens from her relaxed position on the bed beside me. She looks at me sorrowfully.*) They're such a poor lot. Don't waste your precious time, my dear. They're definitely not scholarship material. (*She has* *said this on other visits and refers to the other residents as if they were high school students. She is as confused as any of them but she still has enough remaining insight to know they are 'slow' but not enough to realise that they are as intellectually disabled as she is herself. She feels that she does not belong and tries to make some sense of that. These are companions she would not have chosen if she were able to choose. She rambles on and on as if we are teachers in a school.*)

Eileen: (*Cutting in on her confabulations to bring her back to the things I know give her pleasure. I also realise that she is probably tired.*) Charlotte, I've brought you a little gift. Look. (*I show her the little holy picture of the first Easter morning and it seems to please her.*) Today is Tuesday. On Friday it will be the day of our Lord's crucifixion. Then comes Easter Sunday.

Charlotte: A gift for me. Thank you. Easter… (*She is straining now. It is as if she knows there is something to remember, but she is lost.*)

Eileen: Yes, Charlotte, Easter. I am going to read from the Bible now. (*I read Luke 22:7–20. It is familiar to her and she recites from memory verses 17 and 18. She is softly crying. I take her hands in mine and thought I would ask to pray for us both but before I can do that she picks up my Bible. One of my markers falls out; there is a picture and the first verse of Psalm 23. Charlotte reads it and then completes the psalm from memory. It is a beautiful moment and exactly the right prayer for us. A sharp knock on the door startles us. The door opens.*)

Jean: (*Care home assistant*) Excuse me. Lunch time!

Eileen: Time for me to go, Charlotte. It's lunch time for you. Come, I'll walk to the dining room with you.

Charlotte: Lunch time? Did that girl ring the bell?

Eileen: Lunch time. (*We walk to the dining-room.*) Goodbye for now, Charlotte. Thank you for a very happy visit. I'll come to see you next Tuesday.

Charlotte: Then you must come for lunch. (*She extends her hand and we shake hands very formally.*) So kind of you to call. Thank you.

Eileen: Bless you. And thank you. Goodbye for now, Charlotte.

QUESTIONS FOR DISCUSSION OR REFLECTION

Priests, ministers and pastoral visitors or ministry students could use the above conversation and the following questions for reflection and discussion.

1. What have you learned about Charlotte? Be specific.

2. Identify the use of memory cueing, reality orientation and affirmation of feeling in this verbatim report.

3. What spiritual support was given to Charlotte?

4. Do you think Eileen also received something in this encounter?

5. How could the minister, priest, chaplain or pastoral visitor help Charlotte to maintain a sense of identity for as long as possible?

6. Do you think reading the Bible is a spiritual resource for Charlotte?

7. What non-religious resources would you say, from knowledge gained in this conversation, are a source of spiritual nourishment for Charlotte?

8. Who 'led' the encounter, Charlotte or Eileen?

9. Are there places in this conversation where you would respond differently? Where? Why?

Use of traditional symbols

No one has ever enquired of me what is the one thing above all others which I desire for the people for whom I care and to whom I minister. If they did, I have the answer all ready – I yearn for them to know that God loves them, never forgets them and values the life they live. Of course I know that this is a work of grace. I also know that the Church is meant to be the bearer of God's grace. This surely means that if my hope is ever to be fulfilled we need to find effective new ways to communicate God's love to older people with failing mental powers. We have a long, long way to go.

It is not easy to speak of God to people with dementia because they have little or no memory of the conversation and they cannot keep it focused. In his story of his own journey into Alzheimer's disease, Robert Davis (1989, pp.131–137) is able to give us some assistance and pointers when he shares the changes he experiences at an early stage of the first, or forgetfulness, stage of the disease.

These are some of the difficulties he faces in his experience of God in the cloud of Alzheimer's disease.

- The emotional relationship with God is seemingly destroyed.
- It is very difficult to pray.
- Much of scripture is now unhelpful. The psalms and some of the sayings of Jesus are the exceptions.
- Inability to participate meaningfully in normal congregational worship.
- The sermon can no longer help him. He experiences it as a bewildering jumble of words.
- The modern church music no longer evokes God's presence.

What does Davis tell us of 'helps' to knowing God's loving presence? First he points to the whole of creation. The Psalmist notes:

> The heavens are telling the glory of God; and the firmament proclaims his handiwork. Day to day pours forth speech and night to night declares knowledge.

> There is no speech, nor are there words; their voice is not heard; yet their voice goes out through all the earth, and their words to the end of the world. (Psalm 19:1–4)

Watching National Geographic television programmes helps Robert Davis to find joy and comfort in God's presence. Many who have no formal religion but who are aware of their spiritual needs experience the Creator revealed in creation. The reader may recall the confused woman in a Manchester hospital who was taken to the park.

But Davis also points to the use of symbols. At church on Sunday a young couple gave Robert Davis a beautifully wrapped little parcel. When he opened it he found that it was a picture of Jesus holding up and snuggling a little lamb into his shoulder. Davis claims that this picture changed his whole spiritual outlook at that time, bringing him to his knees so that he cried out his difficulties and implored Jesus to carry him, even as he lovingly carried the lamb in the picture (1989, p.129).

Traditional symbols, used perhaps in new and different ways, can assist those with a dementia illness to sense the loving presence of God with them. This may mean that traditional symbols such as incense, icons, a crucifix, holy pictures, flowers, oil, candles, dance and mime, long used by the Roman

Catholic and Eastern Orthodox traditions and rejected by Protestants at the time of the Reformation, must be brought into use again in the service of those who may now experience God through their senses rather than their intellect. This may not sit well with some of the reformed Churches, but if honestly faced may enrich not only those suffering diminishing intellectual abilities but the whole Church. Robert Davis was a minister in a large evangelical Presbyterian church. It is unlikely that he ever previously saw any need for a little holy picture as an aid to his faith journey.

Attempting to meet the spiritual needs of people with dementia in new and different ways relevant to them is a way of showing love. God's love is perhaps best shown to people with Alzheimer's disease through the love of those close to them. The most important pastoral task of the Church is to help one another grow into the likeness of Christ. Have we the will to engage in prayer for the resources for such service to people within the Body of Christ who are unable to pray for themselves or others?

I can only speak for myself. It is my sense of helplessness and failure, especially my failure to represent the spiritual needs of my people to local leaders of my own tradition, and my inability to achieve very much for those I am given, that sends me to my knees beseeching God's mercy. This is the experience that hammers home to me the lesson that my practical pastoral work is always to be accompanied by the serious work of intercession. It is this experience which binds my heart to the life and service of the Carmelite sisters at Woodhall in West Yorkshire and to the sisters of the Community of the Sacred Name in my own country. Their prayers seem to kneel beside my own poor prayers whenever I am tired and discouraged.

I am humbled over and over again by the fruit of prayer. Sometimes the effects of disease are such that the person desperately needing the assurance of God's love and presence is unable to accept love from those who care for him or her. It is then that I have found it helpful to use a non-threatening symbol. A toy clown can sometimes help to achieve this when the pastor and others are unsuccessful. I found this to be so one day when I visited Tom.

Tom was a sad and silent 81-year-old man, suffering not only second-stage Alzheimer's disease but also a severe depression. Although the staff of the hospital ward gave him respectful quality care and attention, it seemed that nothing could stir him from his dark place within. Tom did not tolerate being touched and would vigorously avoid it. He related to no one among staff or other ward residents and appeared to ignore the few visitors who came to see him. I longed to 'reach' him.

A friend made for me a delightful floppy clown. He is about 50 centimetres long, his middle is a stout oblong wooden block and his head a small plastic ball, shiny white, on which my friend has painted a clown's face. Yellow wool makes a fringe of hair which pokes from his floppy pointed hat with a large multicoloured pom-pom at its pointed end. His suit is red and white: one half plain red, the other half white with large red polka dots. His legs and arms are the empty sleeves and trouser legs of his suit; his hands and feet are large and made of stiff brown vinyl. He is a delightful little fellow, just bursting with personality. I took him with me to visit Tom. Perhaps Tom would relate to the clown, although unable to risk relating to people.

I entered the lounge area of the ward with the clown sitting on my upper forearm and greeted everyone gathered there. I held the clown up high so that everyone could see him, although only a few showed any interest. That is the way it is with people with a dementia illness.

Eileen: Hello, everyone. I'm Eileen. I'm the Methodist minister visiting you here at Red Oak Hospital. I've brought my friend to meet you all. This is Clown. (*I turn to the clown.*)

Clown: (*An unconvincing clown performance by Eileen*) Hi. Hi, everyone. Hello! Hello! (*I manipulate the clown so that he waves to everyone. He then turns to me as if whispering loudly in my ear.*) They don't say anything.

Eileen: I think they're shy.

Clown: Are they? Well tell them I need help. Tell them I've lost my name.

Eileen: (*To the residents*) My little visitor has lost his name. He wants you to help him find his name.

Mary: Hello. (*Her attention has been captured. She is sitting quite close to us. I notice that Tom is sitting beside her with his eyes open but his face wears a dull, passive expression.*)

Clown: She said 'Hello'. (*To Eileen*) Has she got a name?

Eileen: Yes, her name is Mary.

Clown: Hello, Mary, Mary, Mary, Mary, Mary had a little lamb.

Mary: (*She is red and giggling.*) Ooo… It followed her to school one day… Ooo – Ooo – Ooo. (*She giggles with excitement.*)

Clown: … It made the children laugh and play. (*He claps his hands, pleased with himself.*)

Eileen: (*Moving very slowly over to Tom with the clown on her arm*) Hello, Tom. This is my friend, Clown. He had a name once but he lost it.

Clown: Excuse us, Mary. Hi, Eileen. I like this man. What's his name?

Eileen: You ask him yourself. Go on.

Clown: Hey, Mr. What's y' name? (*He stretches out his hand and touches Tom who, surprisingly, does not resist but looks at it and then curls two of his fingers around the clown's hand. The clown tries to disengage but Tom hangs on.*)

Clown: Oh, golly, golly, golly – he's got me. And he won't tell me his name.

Eileen: His name is Tom. (*To Tom*) Clown has lost his name, Tom. Can you help him find his name? Everyone needs a name, Tom. (*While I am speaking I slowly move the clown until it is sitting on Tom's knee. Tom is still holding the clown's hand and I make the clown shake it. Tom shakes hands then, still with impassive face, puts an arm at the clown's back so that it is gently supported on his knee.*)

Tom: (*Very, very quietly*) Tom. Tom.

Clown: (*Claps his hands, going silly with excitement.*) Tom! Tom! Tom! Tiddley pom pom! Tom! Tom! Tom! Tiddley pom pom! Tom! Tom!

Tom: (*Completely oblivious of everyone else, smiles.*) You're a dear wee man.

Eileen: (*To Clown*) You can stay there with Tom, 'dear wee man', while I go to see Mr Ferryman over there. You be a good wee man for Tom, now.

Clown: Yes, Rev. Sure will.

(*I go off to Mr Ferryman, glancing back every little while to see Clown still being gently supported by Tom who seems to be quietly crying. I leave them while I talk to other residents then quietly move back in front of Tom and Clown. I feel Tom take hold of my skirt and I stop and I kneel down by them. Tom's cheeks are wet with tears.*)

Tom: (*Very quietly*) He's Charlie. Charlie.

Eileen: Oh, Tom. He will be so glad you found his name. (*Now to Charlie*) Well, Charlie, you've got it. Tom found your name. Are you happy, Charlie?

Clown: I'll show you. (*He moves as if to kiss Tom on the cheek. I rather expect Tom to draw back. He doesn't. I take Clown, making him do a little jig in the air. As he dances he sings.*) I'm Charlie the Darlie. I'm Charlie, Charlie – Tommy's little Darlie. (*Out we go, Charlie singing and jigging all the way. At the door I turn to look at Tom. His feet are jigging just a little to the clown's singing and he is smiling just a bit. It is a beginning.*)

Charlie is quite shabby these days. He has often accompanied me in my pastoral work and has been a help in many situations. This was especially so with Tom who gradually came out from his locked-in sad self. Of course, he was still very confused and often had difficulty with finding words and then Charlie would find them for him. I do not think he ever remembered Charlie from one visit to the other but he was always pleased to see him. He appeared not to mind when it was time for me to leave, and let Charlie go from him happily. One day when we were leaving, Charlie burst out with 'Hey, Rev., why don't you give Tom a blessing?'

Why not? Very quietly, moving my arms slowly and smoothly, I made the sign of the cross on Tom's forehead and prayed aloud a short blessing. It was the first time I had seen Tom accept another person's touch; I think it indicated that trust was once more growing within him. I believe Charlie had a great deal to do with that. Perhaps a crazy pastor whose dementia friends have taught her to play may have helped, too.

Symbols can be the means of restoring an ability to relate to others. We have learned that relationships with God, self, others and the environment promote spiritual well-being and can enable persons to experience the divine presence. No doubt drugs also helped, even cured Tom's depression. I knew nothing of his treatment. If they did, that also is the grace of God.

Symbols in early awareness, assessment and diagnosis

Recently I have given much thought to developing a pastoral and caring mode with people who have been given a diagnosis of Alzheimer's disease when in its very early first stage. At this phase of the disease they may understand something of the future which faces them as the disease insidiously progresses and memory and other cognitive functions fail, bringing them to even greater loss. I have written in Chapter 1 of the frequency with which I am asked, 'What will happen to my faith when I can no longer remember?' Those who ask this question may know very little of the function of memory but sense that without memory the human spirit, indeed the whole of one's very being, may wither and die.

Since I am asked this question by people who have given little or no attention to the practice of religion as well as those with a sincere and devout faith and sometimes rich spiritual life, we may reasonably assume that the real concern is spiritual rather than religious and indicates a deep anxiety and an intuitive understanding that life is very much more than the salary or welfare benefit arriving regularly into their bank account. These people fear what memory loss and confusion will do to their ability to access the resources they have used over the years to hold them in life's hard places and which have enabled them to give meaning and purpose to their lives. Early awareness and diagnosis provide the possibility of using time early in the disease's progression for the purpose of identifying and sharing the cues which may trigger remote memories, enabling communication, relationships and a sense of community belonging.

After an ecumenical worship occasion for people with dementia, their care givers, families and friends which I had led during National Alzheimer's Awareness Week in New Zealand, I held a casual conversation with a person in the early stages of Alzheimer's disease. I became aware of the importance of using this 'bonus' time in a manner likely to contribute to the person's future quality of life when memory will have deteriorated to the extent that only remote memories can be brought into consciousness. That conversation and others I have had since have alerted me to some of the opportunities inherent in early diagnosis and awareness. Such a mode as I propose may not be suitable for people suffering multi-infarct dementia where there is little pattern and certainly no clearly defined stages in the progress of the dementia.

A person receiving the diagnosis of Alzheimer's disease has much to grieve and the care giver or pastor has the immediate pastoral task of support and consolation while the person grapples with the meaning and purpose of this change in his or her life. This cannot be done sensitively without a sound understanding of the progress and implications of the disease. The pastoral task is further complicated by the difficulties which arise when a family is grieving together but for different reasons. A husband diagnosed with Alzheimer's disease is not only grieving his own future but also the pain and inevitable losses his wife will experience as the disease progresses in him. She, in turn, grieves for her own loss and the losses she fears for her husband.

Such grief, whether directly or indirectly expressed, needs to be recognised, accepted and appropriately processed.

People need someone to journey with them in that; someone who allows them to be. But who can guard them from wreckage on the rocks of the dark waters of grief? – one who knows that grieving takes time but who also understands that this is time to be used for preparation so that the way ahead is less broken and devastating than it might be otherwise. Could it be that the grief work and the preparation of memory cues to guard at least some of the future could be done together? I have engaged in a pastoral work where this appears to be happening. It is much too soon to make any claims at all as to the worth of this pastoral task. Indeed, it may never be possible. All that I do here is describe this work and the premise on which I am building it.

As I see it, the significance of early awareness and diagnosis – and of the patient's understanding the prognosis – lies in the extra time the person has been given before the brain is so seriously damaged as to make it impossible for him or her to contribute to their ongoing well-being. This extra time is an opportunity to plan, to discover memory cues and to consolidate a life-time of personal values. In particular, it is a chance to explore in suffering at least some of the meaning and purpose of a life that is ending in the presence of much cognitive diminishment but still retains a certain integrity.

That basic 'problem' becomes a matter of urgency for the person facing old age and dementia. Is it possible to sustain the meaning of who I have become in this last stage of my life in the circumstances of a dementia illness? Memory function is essential for attempting this task. Anything that can be done to enable the person with dementia to recover the remote memory will assist in meaning formation.

I stated earlier that Frankl (1978) tells us that if the work of meaning formation is thwarted it is possible that a 'noogenic neurosis', the cause of which is a spiritual matter, may result. I propose that if such a neurosis develops in the person with dementia it may exacerbate his or her confusion. If this is correct, then it follows that it is an urgent spiritual and pastoral work to help the person in the early stages of Alzheimer's disease discover, while still able to do so, symbols which may enable others to trigger or cue his remote memories for the work of communication and relationship maintenance, meaning formation and spiritual health as the disease progresses.

I am finding that the mode I use to assist the person to discover his or her symbols for memory cueing in the time ahead is also assisting and providing for the work of grieving. Over a period of time I encourage the person in the early stage of Alzheimer's disease to reminisce – usually with a close family member who is likely to be the future care giver – in order to identify the significant 'moving on in making meaning' places or events in her life and to discover a helpful symbol to express such events. This encourages a lot of helpful reminiscence, talking, crying and sometimes laughter too. We have then put the symbols of these memories, one at a time as we deal with them, into a special small box, and the person is encouraged to take them out between our times together in the company of a family member or an old and trusted friend. The person talks about each symbol and is reminded of their meaning.

One woman found that much meaning was given to her life in the experience of birthing her children. She chose a different symbol for each child and delighted in taking them out, looking at them, and remembering and sharing the memories with significant others. We found that she chose a pink bootie to remind her of the birth of her first child and a long-kept pressed flower from a bouquet brought to her by a joyful husband after the birth of their first son. These symbols are the keys to storehouses of rich and treasured memories and are often beautiful surprises for spouses, children and grandchildren. Hurts are healed, joys and sorrows shared, pride and praise articulated as a family grows very close in their expressions of grief and love and hope. I am confident that families will remind their loved ones journeying deeper into Alzheimer's disease of their past lives, keeping alive and meaningful the significance of who they are for as long as possible.

I move along fairly quickly – because we do not know how long this intentional reminiscence will be possible – to the immediate circumstances of the Alzheimer's disease diagnosis. I encourage the person to talk the feelings out, expressing all the emotions as they surface and spill over. When the person feels ready I will encourage him or her to choose a symbol which expresses what meaning he or she has found in the whole devastating diagnosis and prognosis. This may take several days or even weeks. It is hard, but it seems to me that in seeking this particular symbol the work of acceptance is being completed. Eventually the symbol is chosen and, according to the person's wishes, may be placed in the special memory box. Sometimes the meaning represented by the symbol is shared with close family members present. Sometimes, according to the person's beliefs, I will pray, dedicating the symbols to their special purposes and giving thanks for the unique life they represent.

Our understanding is that the person with Alzheimer's disease will continue to share the memory box often, in the hope that the symbols will continue to be cues for the memories of a human life lived, of values formed, fulfilled and sometimes failed, goals achieved and of those that were put aside, of relationships both rewarding and wounding, of work well done, of joys and sorrows, of those who are loved and have given love, of a life worth living and, most of all, of suffering bravely accepted in a life which in spite of all that is against it dares to claim the grace of God.

Having been, we continue to be, and if the symbols fail in their work of re-mind-ing the forgetful, others will remember for them, keeping their identity safe in the collective memory of their own people.

It is hoped that if a time eventually comes when care is transferred to others, the box of memories will go too, with the meaning of each symbol recorded in a special book that belongs with the box. The professional care giver will be charged and entrusted to use it as a lens through which the confused old person may be perceived and regarded in his or her new home. It is also anticipated that the box will be useful as a family visiting resource.

The power of touch

One cannot read the gospels without being aware of how often Jesus touched people and how often people tried to touch him. It is obvious how important touching was to Jesus. In touching there was healing and power. Robert Davis (1989) experienced touch as a 'strong spiritual resource'. He longed for Jesus to pick him up and 'snuggle me close' (p.63). He also tell us that comforting him in his fear is definitely no longer a matter of reasoning but rather of a 'soft touch and a gentle voice'.

This is of course instinctive to mothers of small children. The language of touch is not dependent on intellectual prowess. In recent times we have seen the advocacy of therapeutic massage for old people and young babies and there are documented studies which indicate the benefits. This is not the task of a pastor, and male pastors will need to decide the extent of touch with which they feel comfortable and safe. Certainly one cannot pastor old people without realising the prevalence of touch deprivation experienced especially by those in professional care. There can be no difficulty in holding and stroking an old person's hand as we sit talking together and in most instances this has a calming effect, especially with mentally frail elderly people.

Sometimes old people clearly indicate their need to be touched, stroked and caressed and the pastor, although witness to the kind of healing which touch appears to evoke, is left wondering exactly what has taken place. What follows is the account of a pastoral encounter with a woman in the assessment unit of a city hospital. Any parish pastor could find himself or herself visiting an elderly parishioner in such a situation.

Mary was difficult for staff to manage, as witness these remarks: 'Can walk – won't walk'; 'Calls out repetitively'; 'Wants to go to bed'; 'Wants this, wants that…'; 'Wants, wants, wants!'; Mary's language became foul, abusive and out of character since she arrived in the ward a week ago. Her life history revealed a strong interest and involvement in religion but she became very aggressive when a priest visited her that morning. Awaiting assessment, she was known to be confused and severely memory-impaired and her family and general practitioner were concerned for her health and safety living, as she had been, by herself. I had not met her before this encounter. She was sitting hunched up, taut, silent and wary. I sat down beside her.

Eileen: Good morning, Mary. May I sit here with you for a while?

Mary: (*Drawing back from me*) Silly old bugger! Silly old bugger! You're a silly old bugger! Silly old bugger! Silly old b –! (*All this is being screamed at me. Mary's face is contorted in what I assume is rage.*)

Eileen: (*Embarrassed but determined not to show it, I am aware that some staff members are amused and others seem anxious. I answer Mary as matter-of-factly as I can.*) How right you are. (*Well, I have to be silly to do this as an unpaid ordained pastor, I think to myself.*)

Mary: You're a bastard! Bastard! Bastard! (*With much feeling and with still louder screaming. I am aware that other patients are very quiet and watching anxiously.*)

Eileen: (*Quietly but firmly*) Now that I am not. Are you really as angry as you sound?

Mary: (*Cuts in*) Want a cup o' tea! (*She fairly spits the words at me. Her body is rigid and her face is strained and red. Her eyes are empty. I am aware that I am no longer embarrassed or afraid. My predominant feeling is of an enormous compassion. I continue very calmly.*)

Eileen: Well, Mary, it is not a cup of tea time. You and I are going to have to wait for that.

Mary: Want a cup o' tea! Want a cup o' tea! (*She is screeching horribly and screaming louder with each word.*)

Eileen: (*Calmly, firmly, and with authority*) Stop screaming at me. I don't like it. (*I am aware that I feel confidently, sympathetically, in charge. Mary looks at me for the first time. I gently take her poor mis-shapen hands in mine, half expecting her to snatch them away, but she doesn't.*) My name is Eileen. Hello, Mary.

Mary: Silly old bugger. Silly older bugger. (*Softer now, as I gently stroke her hands.*)

Eileen: I like your name. Mary is a pretty name. Mary?

Mary: Mary, bastard.

Eileen: Mary is an upset old lady. I'm sorry. I'm really sorry you are so distressed, Mary. (*Now she carries my hand to her forehead and I softly stroke and caress her.*)

Mary: (*Jerking herself and beginning with a whining kind of screaming*) Want to go to bed! Want to go to bed! (*Getting louder and louder*)

Eileen: (*Patiently, firmly*) It's not night time, Mary. We go to bed at night. (*I become aware that I have stopped stroking her forehead as Mary moves my hand to begin again. I do so. I am aware that I am paying attention to all that is happening to Mary. I am paying attention from a place in my body – it seems like my gut.*)

Mary: (*After some moments of silence during which her body relaxes a little*) Daddy – Daddy – My Daddy – Gone – Dead. (*In anguish*) Daddy, my Daddy.

Eileen: (*I wait a few seconds before speaking. I am aware that something profoundly significant is happening.*) Poor Mary. You are very upset. We do care about you. (*She has closed her eyes and her stiff body softens and begins to relax as I continue to stroke and caress her forehead. We sit quietly like this for some minutes. The ward seems unusually quiet. I am aware that I, too, am relaxed and peace-filled.*)

Mary: (*Very softly*) Our Father, who art in heaven, hallowed be thy name... (*She softly, slowly prays all the Lord's Prayer. I pray softly with her. Mary is really quite beautiful, relaxed and quiet. Her eyes are closed.*)

Eileen: (*I sit with Mary quietly for some minutes. She opens her eyes and almost smiles.*) I'll be back, Mary. (*I get up to leave.*) Bless you, now.

As I moved to another patient I passed one of the ward nurses who quietly remarked, 'We don't have pills that can do that, Eileen.' Indeed we don't.

At home that evening as I wrote up my verbatim notes I reflected deeply and marvelled at the strong sense of peace that finally settled on Mary and myself and, it seemed, upon the whole of the ward day room. My report indicated that I had used the tools of orientation: I had continually brought Mary to the reality of the day room, that is, tea was served at set times, bed and sleep are for the night hours, and I am not a bastard although I may well be 'silly'. This is what I call negative orientation and I usually try not to use it, that is I actively denied Mary's seeming reality at these points. However, further on in the encounter I was able to state simply the present reality: I affirmed the reality of Mary's name, I reflected back to her the feelings of anger and inner turmoil which were real and in doing so I affirmed her feelings. It is possible that memory cueing was used through the caressing of Mary's forehead (touching). It does seem to me that this triggered a remote memory which prompted Mary's recitation of the Lord's Prayer. I was also aware of the paying attention that seems to take place from my gut and I welcomed that mystery.

Using self-included humour

During my ministry to people with a dementia illness, especially Alzheimer's disease, I have developed an understanding and appreciation of humour as a resource for spiritual well-being. Because the person with Alzheimer's disease usually occupies a different reality from others, the opportunity to use this resource is infrequent. But it is worthwhile being alert to the opportunities. Of course we must never laugh at confused people, only with them, and it is always best if the humour includes ourselves. There have been a few occasions like the incident with Kay mentioned earlier when the situation has been so funny that I have not been able to keep myself from laughing. I hope such laughter is always kindly. The risk of hurting is real and I try not to take such risks, saving my laughter to share with a supervisor or other trusted person. My ability to see the humour even in what looks like doom and gloom is a sign of my own growing spiritual maturity.

I was late for my usual weekly service with a little group of eight Christians in a care home. Each is a faithful disciple of Christ. They are all experiencing various degrees of confusion and memory loss for various different reasons. I had been with this group each week for a little over twelve months. They always appear to enjoy this weekly worship although they forget me and the worship from one week to the next – probably, indeed, before I have reached the gate.

On this occasion all are sitting around a battered table used mostly by the activities organiser. This woman is a Christian and it was her initiative with management which first brought me here. She had let me know of the two Methodists in the group and her perception that they needed pastoral care and worship opportunities. I appreciate that she judges it important to share worship with this little group.

Eileen: (*Entering the small room we use*) Hello, everyone. I'm sorry I'm so late.

Betty: Are you late?

Eileen: Yes, I am, Betty. (*I greet each person by name, shaking hands. They forget who I am but do seem to find me a 'familiar friend' and most reach out to embrace me and be embraced.*)

Eileen: (*Slowly but naturally, making eye contact with each person*) I'm Eileen. I'm the Methodist minister. I come here every week on Tuesday morning. Today is Tuesday. We are at Hartland House nursing home. You live here. I've come to bring you the love of the Church and to worship God with you.

Allan: Yes Eileen. (*When I have reminded Allan of my name he always uses it to address me. Names are important to people with dementia illness.*) That's good. I used to go to church...forget...

Eileen: You used to go to the church in Addington, Allan. Betty was a local preacher at Ohoka, Margaret went to St Margaret's at Oakfields and Sam went to St Ninian's in Beachside. You all used to go to your own church. Now that you live at Hartland House we have church here. We are the church in this place.

Dorothy: (*Slowly as, the most advanced in her illness, she struggle to find the words*) Church. Church. We sing.

Eileen: Yes, we sing, Dorothy. We will sing some hymns. Look, here is my tape recorder. I'm putting the tape in like this... (*We are interrupted by a young woman who wants to clean the room. Helen, the activities organiser, explains that we are a little late with our church service this morning.*)

Eileen: I'm sorry to delay your schedule because I was late. I drove my car out of the garage with plenty of time to get here and found it felt funny and wouldn't steer properly. The front tyre was flat. That tyre was flat as a pancake.

Betty: Oh dear. Flat as a pancake.

Eileen: Yes, Betty, as flat as a pancake. That flat tyre made me late.

Margaret: What did you say when you saw it? (*An unusual response; people with failing mental powers caused by a dementia illness do not normally ask questions related to a previous statement. I didn't think of that at the time and answer very quickly, laughing and shaking my finger with mock sternness.*)

Eileen: I'm not telling you.

Margaret: (*Laughing knowingly*) Oh. Oh. I like that… It makes you one of us. (*This was a moment of pure delight, teasing, puckish fun, a moment of happy mutuality as we shared this spontaneous humour which is rarely possible with confused people.*)

Betty: I like it when we laugh.

Margaret: You're just like us. (*Still laughing, full of delight and wagging her finger at me*)

Allan: (*Looking puzzled and perhaps a bit put out*) I want to sing. (*I get up and go to hug Margaret who hugs me too. Then I light our candle and place the cross beside it in the centre of the table.*)

Eileen: God is here.

All: God is always here.

Eileen: God is with us.

All: God is always with us. (*After a little silence*)

Eileen: Now we'll sing 'What a friend we have in Jesus'. (*We continued with worship*).

Questions for discussion or reflection

1.   On what basis were the pastor and Margaret relating?

2.   Can you think of incidents in the gospels where Jesus used humour?

Such an encounter cannot be planned. It will happen spontaneously if it happens at all. However, the attitudes and values of the pastor are important for the healing quality of any pastoral encounter. The key word is respect: for diversity, simplicity, personhood, the present moment, mutuality, relatedness, paying attention, prayer, mystery and, above all, the God of infinite surprises.

Spiritual care of the person near to death

Dying begins at birth. This is a positive not a morbid truth. The whole of life is a preparation for our dying. Death and bereavement are times of enormous spiritual power. To accompany people who are dying on this last part of their life journey is to make a hard and holy pilgrimage. The advent words which live year after year in the memory are those from the book of Isaiah: 'In the wilderness prepare the way of the Lord. Make straight in the desert a highway for our God' (Isaiah 40:3).

I am familiar with death. Even so, at the beginning of my ministry to people with failing mental abilities that was not enough. I recall clearly when the advent message pierced my consciousness with insight and gave shape to my caring. The prophet's words were invocation to a mind-picture of the impending arrival of a great and noble ruler who desires that those who are in any kind of distress be given comfort. The road over which this one must travel is to be cleared. No rocks or holes or bends or narrowness can be left to impede the way. So I see myself as a 'road-mender' in what often feels like a wilderness place – the lonely desert place of seeming, but only seeming, nothingness. Spiritual caring is the removing of obstacles that are in the way of the God who comes. '"Comfort, O comfort my people," says your God' (Isaiah 40:1). This is a message to exiles in preparation for their return. It is not just for those who are chosen among the dying ones but for everyone.

How can we transform the message of the one who comes into a reality of caring for those who can no longer remember? In a way the whole of this book is an attempt to share with those who care a way to do that. It offers a way to remove the obstacles to bringing courage, strength and all that is associated with that wonderful word 'comfort' – the familiar, a relaxation and warmth, cosiness and homeliness. Spiritual care for dying and bereaved people is a work in the wilderness of the place where people are. It is often done in a desert terrain of loss, confusion and distressing forgetfulness. To comfort dying people with declining mental powers and to make straight the path along which God comes to them is the privileged work of a spiritual care giver.

It is not just the work of the pastor, priest or chaplain. The obstacles are many and varied – physical, emotional and spiritual – and they require an holistic approach. Doctors, nurses, care givers, families, friends, gardeners, cooks, cleaners, post-women, music makers and story-tellers. The reader may wish to turn back to Chapter 3 to read again the case stories of May, Jim and Charlotte.

Dying people need love, reconciliation, acceptance and the deep sense of being valued and respected in their vulnerability so that they may be endowed with dignity and integrity. They need an affirmation of God's presence. This can be conveyed through the memory cueing of familiar prayers, hymns, scriptures, liturgy, absolution, anointing and the sacrament of holy communion.

Different Christian traditions – as well as different faith traditions and cultures such as Judaism or Islam – all have their own particular rituals and cultural customs in the presence of death and grief. Responsible care means institutional management will find appropriate ways and personnel to provide for these.

Although it is not usual in my own Christian tradition, I often use the practice of anointing the dying person. I find this beautiful ritual to be particularly relevant to the needs of a person whose awareness and knowing do not come from the intellect but through the five senses, particularly smell and touch. With perfumed oil I make the sign of the cross on the person's forehead and the palms of both hands, with the following two prayers, adapted with permission from *A New Zealand Prayer Book* (Collins 1989):

> (Name) I anoint you with this holy oil. Receive Christ's forgiveness. The power of the Saviour who redeems you flow through your mind and body, lifting you to that peace and inward strength which our Lord's victory over the powers of chaos and darkness has won for all his people. Amen.

After the anointing I will offer a short and simple prayer such as this:

> God our healer, keep us aware of your presence. Support us with your power. Comfort us with your protection. Give us strength and establish us in your presence. Amen.

Or this:

> Lord Jesus, let the peace of your presence enfold (Name) and those who love and care for her/him. Amen.

Sometimes the concept of anointing is too strange for some families but they believe that comfort will be given their dying loved one if a blessing is given.

For those who are not Christian believers I sometimes suggest that perfumed oil is used to massage hands or temples and forehead. A family member or care giver can do this as a sensory expression of caring, loving and comforting. Fine clean bed linen, flowers, candles and music also help to show love and bestow dignity. Ministry to the dying person with failing mental powers brings us to a sense of our own poverty. Very often there is nothing to do but be. God asks his disciples to watch and wait while God, too, prays. It is enough. Grace comes, gently, filling the moments as a costly perfume fills a room with its essence. Into the heart comes an absolute certainty. All is well.

More detailed guidance for ministers and family carers in visiting those in care will be found in Appendixes 8 and 9.

Summary

Although many, including the ordained minister, may provide for a variety of pastoral needs, it is the particular call and responsibility of the ordained person to provide nurture for the spiritual well-being of the person with this devastating disease as he journeys home in his own unique cloud of unknowing. The challenge is to find a way which upholds the person who has limited ability to remember or organise his own thinking.

The two bright stars of hope which will encourage the pastor and care giver in the pastoral task are these.

- The ability to feel and respond to feeling remains intact in the person with Alzheimer's disease long after he or she has lost the ability to understand. We know also that 'small islands' of ability remain in the brain and these should be acknowledged and used. We do not know about the predictability of appropriate feeling responses of people suffering other types of dementia.

- The remote memory can be cued sometimes well into the progressive stages of Alzheimer's disease. Those with responsibility for the spiritual well-being of people with dementia must develop approaches to ministry that involve greater initiative from the pastor and care giver. It is the responsibility of the ordained pastor to provide the initiative for training lay pastors who can assist in this ministry. Most lay people cannot do it alone without training.

Suggestions for reflection following the verbatim accounts of actual pastoral conversations or encounters (given above) illustrate the principles and tools available for effective relevant pastoral caring. These are: an initial orientation to present reality, an affirmation of feelings, cueing of remote memories, the use of symbols and different ways of thinking and relating, humour and responsible touching. It is essential to have a genuine respect for the disabled person which is independent of our culture's high regard for 'usefulness' and 'doing' rather than the sacredness of 'being'. It is a matter of justice that the person with dementia is remembered, valued and included within the life of the faith community.

Although the need to find meaning and purpose in life usually leads a person to a belief system, faith in the transcendent other and the practice of a religion, this is not always so. Intelligent and loving attempts should be made to connect the non-religious person with the benevolent source or sources of his or her spiritual well-being with as much integrity as for those of religious faith.

The person of Christian faith can be assured over and over again that he or she is loved by God and can never be separated from the One who never forgets us.

Above all, the Christian care giver and pastor need never feel alone or powerless. We have available to us a work of intercessory prayer for all our people's needs and griefs. The privilege of bringing our people into relation with the divine love is a costly work. It is a burden – but it is also the eagle's wings on which the weary care giver and pastor may be carried.

6

Caring for the Care Givers

But Moses' hands grew weary; so they took a stone and put it under him, and he sat on it. Aaron and Hur held up his hands, one on one side, and the other on the other side; so his hands were steady until the sun set. (Exodus 17:12)

It takes a saint to do this kind of work. (Oral report from a care giver)

By the year 2020 it has been forecast in the United States of America one half of all deaths will occur after 80 years of age, and there are no reasons why this should not happen in New Zealand... In New Zealand we now have smaller families, often spread geographically. Most families do provide care for their older members when and if it is required. Unfortunately, the families commonly do not get the support they need from the formal domiciliary support services. (Koopman-Boyden 1993, pp.68–69)

The situation described above also applies in the UK and many other countries. As Alzheimer's disease and other related dementia illnesses progress, people with these disorders become increasingly dependent upon family. The presence of a family care giver is one of the main factors preventing the institutionalisation of dependent older people. By far the greatest number of people with these illnesses (80%) are cared for at home – their own or that of a close family member. Most will be cared for by a spouse, who is likely to be 70 years plus, or a daughter who may also be caring for little children or teenagers. The caring period, unlike that of other terminal illness such as cancer, will go on for many years, gradually claiming more and more of the care giver's time and energy as the disease relentlessly progresses into increasing deterioration. Some care givers will be faced with difficult-to-manage, energy-sapping kinds of behaviours.

Some of these difficult behaviours could be: wanting to be up and active at night and wanting to sleep during the day, wandering, aggression, inappropriate sexual behaviours, incontinence and inability to stop asking the same question over and over again. Eventually a time comes when one person alone can no longer sustain the 24-hour care necessary for the loved one's well-being. The painful process of transferring care to professional care givers in a care home or hospital must be undertaken.

If family care givers and their loved ones at home are to receive pastoral and spiritual care, it will have to come from the faith community. However, churches can (and do) so easily lose touch with care givers as well as people with a dementia illness. One couple, caring for the wife's elderly, very confused, physically frail mother told me they found it impossible to meet their own need to be part of their faith community's worship together and now went to church alone on alternate Sundays. So unaware of the situation was the presbyter (and people) of their church that no one discerned that this couple very much missed worshipping together. Worse, on one occasion each was asked to read the Scripture lessons and prepare the prayers of intercession on the same Sunday.

Anne Opie, in her book *Caring Alone* (1991) provides verbatim interview reports of the primary care givers' experiences of caring in the home for family members with Alzheimer's disease or – less frequently – multi-infarct types of dementia. One conversation is particularly sad. An elderly man, 76 years old, caring alone for his wife with Alzheimer's disease, when asked about social contacts – possibly the couple's church community – replied that although he was connected with his church from an early age and was an elder for over 45 years, they now experienced no contact or support from their church.

The Church's ministry to Elderly Confused People, the work I have pioneered in New Zealand, commissioned a survey of clergy and church women's groups in my city. The unpublished report of 1994 indicates that the majority of priests and ordained ministers who responded knew of no one in their congregations who suffered from Alzheimer's disease or any other type of dementia and they knew of no one in their parish who was a primary care giver. Yet the majority of women in the Women's Fellowships of those same parishes indicated that they knew of both sufferers and family care givers.

In caring for my mother I also experienced the Church's lack of awareness of the nature of dementia illness. I am sometimes told of a particularly damaging situation which develops in this way:

> Mrs Jones, a widow, lives in parish A. and is a devoted member of her church. Recently, after competent assessment, she has received a diagnosis

of early dementia, probably Alzheimer's disease. Her daughter Jane is a member of the church in parish B. Naturally she is very worried and concerned for her mother, so Jane phones the mother's minister in parish A and tells him of her concern for her mother over some time, and the recently received diagnosis, and then asks him to visit her mother. The presbyter does so a few days later and, knowing very little about Alzheimer's disease, expects to greet a very sick woman. Instead, Mrs Jones, although unable to remember his name, does recognise his clerical collar. Mrs Jones knows how to talk to the minister, and does so quite capably for the fifteen to twenty minutes of his visit. The presbyter leaves bewildered, concluding that both Jane and the doctor must be mistaken. Later that day he phones Jane and tells her kindly but firmly that there is nothing wrong with her mother, certainly nothing to cause Jane such anxiety, and then he confidently advises her not to worry and to seek another doctor's opinion. With a kindly goodnight he puts down the telephone and hurries off to his church's finance committee meeting. This good man has no thought of Jane who, in tears, is answering another call. This call is the tenth she has had from her mother that day and she is complaining out of her forgetfulness and confusion that no one visits her, 'not even the minister'.

These are hurtful and damaging incidents. Added to the care giver's already heavy burdens these hurts can settle like a lump of lead on the heart and shake the care giver's faith and confidence in the Church as a caring community. Although her faith in God may not be, the meaning and purpose of her own and her loved one's suffering are even harder to discern.

Such stories reveal not an apparent hardness of heart but rather a need for education in this area of pastoral care. There are more intellectually impaired old people living in the community than the number living in care homes or hospitals, and with a policy of care in the community this trend is likely to continue and increase. Considering the global demographic trend of an ageing population, it is possible that in the future some couples will have no one, or at the most only one sibling, to share in the caring of 12 old, and perhaps seriously dependent, people: four parents and eight grandparents. Such a situation is impossible to grapple with without the help of others in the community, some of whom will be just as burdened. Undoubtedly, Christian people and the Church will be a part of this community assistance to care givers in all kinds of need, including advocacy.

Although a healthy approach to care giver community support must necessarily be holistic, it is my intention to concentrate on the spiritual dimension of pastoral caring for care givers since there are resources providing for physical, emotional and social needs available through other community organisations such as the Alzheimer's Society. The Church, unlike other institutions, exists primarily to meet spiritual need. Nevertheless, the spiritual is grounded in the ordinary and I shall point the reader in that direction as well as towards the mystery of the transcendent and immanent God. We will also explore the implications of the practice of religion by those whose sustaining source of spiritual health is found in their faith beliefs and religious practices. Although we may separate body and soul, for the purposes of discussing one of these dimensions the two, in Judeo–Christian thinking, belong together and effective pastoral work embraces the whole.

Pastors cannot help the care giver towards spiritual health without an understanding of the specific situation of the care giver and of how this context may impact upon spiritual needs.

Care-givers of people with Alzheimer's disease and related dementias face:

- social isolation
- grief
- insufficient time for self, family and friends
- the unresolved heavy physical labour of care-giving
- financial burden
- loss of hobbies and the opportunity for the pursuit of new interests, learning and realisation of long-term goals in retirement
- career disruptions and lost promotion opportunities
- anger, guilt and denial.

The affective context of care givers

Research (Wilson 1989) indicates that the most critical factors influencing a care giver's ability to sustain his or her role without feelings of victimisation by family and community are:

- the quality of the care giver's relationship with the dependent person
- the attitude of the care giver to his or her role.

If these conditions are positive, care givers seem not to be overwhelmed by the stress and constancy of their task. The greater the emotional distancing between care giver and the cared-for person the greater the sense of burden and resentfulness.

Anne Opie (1991) proposes that there are four affective positions which care-givers occupy. She has labelled these commitment, obligation, dissociation and repudiation.

1. *Commitment.* This is the position adopted by care givers who are most able to accept their family member's disability and maintain a positive sense of relationship.

2. *Obligation.* This describes the affective response of relatives whose caring is motivated primarily as the result of trying to live up to other people's expectations of their obligation to care. Their relationship with their confused relative is more distant than that of a care giver positioned within commitment.

3. *Dissociation.* Opie (1991) uses this word to describe an even greater degree of distancing from the confused person.

4. *Repudiation.* This is the most powerful affective position. It describes a relationship in which the care giver is able to affirm very little positive warmth towards the confused person being cared for and where the caring is experienced as distasteful and burdensome.

None of these emotional positions is gender specific. Sons as well as daughters may undertake the responsibilities of care giver because of genuine commitment, rather than grudgingly because of family and community expectation. It is very easy to judge harshly those care-givers who find their role a distasteful burden. No one has the right to do that, least of all the person without any personal experience of dementia illness in a close family member.

Pastors need to know that, according to a research project undertaken in the US, (Pratt, Schmall and Wright 1985), care givers separate potential sources of support into those who have and those who have not travelled the road themselves. Certainly I felt this in the early days of establishing a ministry among older confused people and their care givers. Initially I was accepted by care givers because I had been there. My understanding came out of my own experience. Although it was also informed by study, that seemed hardly to matter to them. Consequently the pastor who listens attentively to the care giver's experience is likely to win confidence and be of real assistance.

All care givers, regardless of their emotional positioning, may experience varying degrees of resentment, pain, fear and, most of all, loss. It is wise for a pastor to acknowledge how fine is the line separating abuse from caring love in many difficult situations and to approach the subject of abuse with honesty and sturdy compassion. Abuse is more often a sign that the care giver needs more support and practical help rather than one of callous disregard. It should be met with strong although compassionate solutions.

In terms of the strategies which may assist care givers to cope with the burdens of care-giving, the same research project showed that care givers rated spiritual support before friends and neighbours and before community services as their most helpful coping strategy (Pratt, Schmall and Wright 1985). Families who use spiritual support as a strategy for coping value the visits and empathy of clergy, supporting prayer, being able to attend their church's worship, taking part in church activities. They especially appreciate men's or women's fellowship groups and small bible study groups which explore the biblical models of caring.

One elderly man who described his care-giving work in the metaphor of a kind of exile was helped enormously by rediscovering these verses in Isaiah:

> Can a woman forget her nursing child, or show no compassion for the child of her womb? Even these may forget, yet I will not forget you. See, I have inscribed you upon the palms of my hands. (Isaiah 49:15–16a)

Likening his own cut-off life to the captivity of the people of Judah and their exile in foreign Babylon, he looked for God in his own situation and was able to say to me one day, out of the inspiration he had found in the exile story:

> You know Eileen, not every day, but on enough days I can say, and mean it too – and I tell her, 'Joyce my old darling,' I say, 'seems like they've all forgotten you and me, but not quite you know. Our names are written on God's hands. How about that? You and me on God's hands.'
>
> Well, Eileen, things don't get any better, you know that. But it really matters what you use for the measuring. I got to thinking about that. I said to myself, 'Look here, Lionel, old man, do you believe that God forgot our Lord hanging on that bloody cruel cross? You do not, Lionel,' I said, 'no way.' And really, Eileen, I don't care a damn – not really – who the hell forgets about us, 'cause Joyce and me are on God's hands. Good God, Joyce and me on God's hands!

An unconventional statement of faith? Nowhere near the Nicene creed for beauty of language. But as natural and honest and strong, hard and beautiful as crystal, cut to reflect every ray of light.

As far as I know at the time of writing, no one in New Zealand except Anne Opie (1991) has researched family care giver needs and attitudes as care givers themselves rate them. My feeling is that if this American research were done in New Zealand or in the UK our understanding of spiritual support would be quite different from that in the North American research where there is still a largely church-going society. It is as well to remember that although a Kiwi care giver may be more likely to request time out from caring for a long walk in the park or countryside than for time to attend church worship, both are authentic means of spiritual renewal. The human spirit may reach out to the divine Spirit seeking renewal and refreshment in the New Zealand bush or in a church service.

We will be in good company in either place: which is not to say I believe that Sunday church worship does not matter. It does: we Christians will never reach our true destination pushing on alone. Just as our great mountain climbers needed companions if they were to reach Mt Everest's summit, so we human beings will never reach our 'spiritual Everest' without the company of others. Each Sunday, whether inclined to or not, we must make it to the pew and do our best for each other and God, in spite of the sometimes strange antics that take place in church. When pastoring the tired care giver, however, pastors should show a little mercy and encourage the care giver who so wishes to listen to 'the trees clapping their hands' (Isaiah 55:12), 'the forests singing for joy' (Psalm 96:12b) and 'the heavens telling the glory of God' (Psalm 19:1) while our 'mountains skip like rams and the hills like lambs' (Psalm 114:4).

Many care givers do ask for prayer or will gratefully accept it if it is offered during a visit. Some would like a home mass or service of holy communion with family, friends and neighbours. Religion as a spiritual resource provides confidence in re-framing problems. It is advantageous for the care giver to be able to discern and choose the least negative option from what the care giver perceives to be negative choices, for example, 'Do I put her into a nursing home now or do I give her more time at home with me and burn out?' Spiritual support of this nature will often open up the way by which the care giver begins to ask the critical questions of his or her situation, leading to the discovery of meaning and purpose in the undeserved suffering of all who must bear the losses inherent in dementia illness, and so continue as Lionel did without resentment and soul-destroying bitterness.

Those care givers who have come to the place of transferring the care of their loved ones to professional care givers in a residential setting continue to carry the same sense of burden and stress as before. It appears to be an easing of the physical burdens of exhaustion and psychological crowding that makes a difference to the care giver's health. However, for spouses there are the stresses of living alone. In this circumstance care givers need the same level of pastoral support as when they cared as the primary care giver at home. Care givers need to know that they do not have to face their problems alone. Some community resources are available. It is part of good care-giving to utilise those which will make a positive difference to well-being. The informed pastor can offer help with information of community services.

Implications for ministry

The presbyter or pastoral care giver's calling in the situation we are considering is to mediate the presence of God to people with Alzheimer's disease or other primary dementia and their families, and to lead their congregations in providing communities of practical support and concern for them. As the people of God, each congregation is charged with caring over the long haul even although they may receive little in return. How they do so will have an important impact on the spiritual health of family carers.

Earlier in this book I identified three essential factors for the maintenance of spiritual health and well-being: a sense of identity; right relatedness with God, self, others and the environment; and a sense that life has meaning and purpose. We need now to reflect on how these factors relate to the work of a care giver.

Sense of identity

My own experience of caring for my mother generated intense spiritual yearning and heightened spiritual awareness although I have since discovered that this yearning is common to almost all care givers whatever their circumstances and previous spiritual awareness. I found little understanding of this at that time. However, I had discovered this enormous spiritual sensitivity and yearning within myself when my husband died suddenly while still in his forties. As I grieved my own and my sons' loss, I found for myself resources to assuage the yearning and spiritual hunger which drew me nearer to the meaning and purpose of a life now drastically changed.

I found this spiritual help in books and discovered the writings of people such as Sheila Cassidy, Allan Jones, Thomas Merton, Teilhard de Chardin, Kenneth Leech, Constance Fitzgerald, Rosemary Haughton and many others. Only very seldom does the Church, through the pastor or its members, recognise this most fertile ground of faith and spiritual growth and minister to it from out of its own rich store of spiritual treasure. Its servants seem not to realise that to minister to this spiritual awareness may be a witness of the transforming power of the divine spirit.

To ignore this spiritual sensitivity is sad because within the yearning is a big question: 'Who am I now?' Grace and previous life experience led me to an even deeper understanding of myself as 'child of God', with a strong inner connectedness to the whole of creation which, no matter what my present circumstances, could not be taken from me. I understood that my essential identity was my God-given 'personhood'. Even so, the days were so crowded with so many roles: mother, friend, teacher, gardener, cook and laundress, comforter, administrator, poetry lover, story-teller, listener, and – hardest to accept – no longer daughter, but mother for my parents.

Some days all these pieces of my identity became like coloured pieces of paper flying in the winds of cold change. Many care givers have told me of their own almost identical experience of threatened identity.

What would help in this threatened loss of personal identity? Anything that reminded and affirmed the care giver's place in the community and in the body of Christ, the Church. In my tradition rarely these days in public worship are we given the opportunity to make a corporate affirmation of our faith by reciting one of the great creeds of the Church. Oh yes, I know that some modern men and women have difficulty with both language and concepts. But in this act of traditional affirmation, who I am and where I stand is, for me, made clear once more. I stand with others in a great chain of people extending through the years, into the future and across the nations. All share the same belonging and relationship. Each one, although one of many, is a unique loved child of the creator God. The liturgical act of affirmation is more than the words. It is my spirit and the spirits of all the others of all the ages reaching out to the Divine Spirit in order to connect with the meaning and purpose of our living and proclaim for each other who we really are – God's children.

The spiritual well-being of the care giver is nourished when:

- the role of care giver is given positive affirmation by the pastor and church family which names care-giving as an act of ministry, a vocation

- in a liturgical and corporate act we affirm our Christian belief and know ourselves as members of a mysterious body which is more than the sum total of all of us

- the church organises pastoral care to include giving care givers the opportunity to attend the worship of the people of God by organising a regular sitter service. This need not be every Sunday but should be discussed with the care giver

- a pastoral care ministry makes it possible for the care giver to remain involved in the Church's fellowship groups

- the presbyter is a person of intercessory prayer, acquainted with the needs of his or her people

- a sensitive pastor is aware of identity needs and discerns ways of affirming identity relevant to particular people. For example, a care giver who has given up his or her career identity in enforced early retirement will perhaps appreciate conversation which indicates a respect for, and interest in, a previous career, work skills and achievements. It may feel to the care giver that this part of self is unacknowledged and forgotten. Such feelings add to some care givers' sense of low self-esteem. Validating the existence of difficult and seemingly unacceptable feelings will foster coping. Feelings are valid and someone who listens to them without judgement is a blessing

- occasional, although regular opportunities are made available for the care giver to indulge in a hobby, craft or particular interest. These will help the care giver maintain identity and can be arranged for by a church organising a sitting service or just the informal offer of a friend to 'hold the fort' for a couple of hours. Time can also be given as gift by preparing food for heating and eating.

A positive relatedness

The care giver of a person with a primary dementia is likely to experience many strains in various relationships as a result of such demanding caring and its prolonged nature. These strains occur in relationships with God, with one's own self, with others and with the environment.

RELATIONSHIP WITH GOD

The role of care giver may severely test the care giver's relationship with God. Some care givers are angry with God and may question why and how God could allow this thing to happen to their loved one. They need assurance that anger is natural. An insightful pastor may find it helpful to offer some expressions of anger and complaint addressed to God by the psalmists and some of the prophets.

Listen to Jeremiah:

> Oh, Lord God of hosts, I did not sit in the company of merrymakers, nor did I rejoice; under weight of your hand I sat alone, for you had filled me with indignation. Why is my pain unceasing, my wound incurable, refusing to be healed? Truly, you are to me like a deceitful brook, like waters that fail. (Jeremiah 15:17–18)

A paraphrase might read: 'Lord I've done the decent thing because you asked me, you stirred me up. I suffer because I'm on your side and you don't seem to care a damn. I'm hurt! Very hurt! You are about as useful to me as a liar. You, who should be my life. You have failed me!' That's anger! Even so, Jeremiah is not cursed. Rather, God tenderly replies:

> I will make you to this people a fortified wall of bronze; they will fight against you, but they shall not prevail over you, for I am with you to save and deliver you. (Jeremiah 15:20)

And now this expression of vengeful wicked anger from the Israelites in exiled captivity, brought upon themselves by their own deliberate turning from Yahweh and covenant:

> O daughter Babyon, you devastator! Happy shall they be who pay you back what you have done to us! Happy shall they be who take your little ones and dash them against the rock! (Psalm 137:8–9)

Shocking, murderous anger! Yet this psalm was not excluded from the canon, although most would hesitate to use verse nine in public worship. It is frightening, terrible.

Anger, however, is a feeling, and feelings in themselves are neither good nor bad. It is what we do with anger that carries a judgement. Obviously it is wrong to hurt people with our own anger. But somehow our anger must be grounded, turned into some kind of physical energy. Otherwise it turns in upon us and we may become depressed. Unless the pastor is appropriately qualified I do not advise counselling but a pastor, friend or family member may be sufficiently strong to listen as the anger is spilled out, perhaps aimed at the undeserving, and absorbed by the listener as an act of ministry. Anger can be productive of change. If properly channelled it can provide energy to help the care giver seek creative and positive ways to change or modify particular situations, the source of the anger against God. I have found that listening with 'gut attention' and acceptance helps the care giver ground the anger. It is taken seriously.

Anger is often dispersed in the commitment to specific action.

RELATIONSHIP WITH SELF

The care giver's anger and consequent guilt has the power to disturb his or her healthy relationship with self. Quietness, a time and suitable place for prayer, reflection and recollection are good resources for restoring friendship with oneself. One care giver told me of the bliss of spending half an hour in a friend's spa pool – mind and body sufficiently relaxed for her to reflect and pray through several matters and discern a positive way ahead.

RELATIONSHIPS WITH OTHERS

The stresses and strains of care giving can drastically disturb the care giver's relationship with those he or she loves – family and friends, and the cared-for person. Tensions and irritation are often the result of spending many hours together at home without the stimulation of others and their ideas. I find walking, loved one and care giver together, is a fine way to bring back joy and balance which iron out the wrinkles of irritation. Gardening together also helps if the person being cared for is physically fit. A change of scene is a restorer of relationship; sometimes the pastor or some other qualified parish person can help facilitate this.

Recalling the healing and peace – even hope – I found in walking with a wise and thoughtful brother-in-law who initiated these walks in the weeks following my husband's sudden death, I began walking with my mother, who was amazingly fit. We enjoyed the gardens in the near neighbourhood and often particular flowers or shrubs would cue her memory so that we could talk together happily in the present, by way of the past. We often walked in the park or botanical gardens and took off our shoes to feel the warm sand between our toes as we strolled by the sea in summer. We both returned to the house pleasantly tired, emotionally and spiritually renewed.

Others tell me that they also find a togetherness, free from tensions and irritability, in physical activity, especially walking. My mother would hold my hand as we walked, just as once, as a child, I placed my hand in hers for confidence and security. Sometimes as we walked she would talk of her mother who had died when she was a girl of 16 years. And sometimes she confused me with my grandmother or her mother. But walking was always a happy time. Those walks are a good memory. As time goes by and the confusion increases, it becomes more and more difficult to find a true togetherness, but walking together is something that can happen for as long as the loved one is mobile. It may continue on if a wheelchair is available and the care giver can learn to walk beside it.

Isolation from peers, friends and associates, and living constantly with someone whose reality is, for the greater part of time, not that of the care giver, can erode not only physical and emotional well-being but also spiritual well-being. When this is allowed to continue the care giver may find it difficult to relate to others. She may become distant or irritable with other family members, friends and well-intentioned visitors from the church, and so become locked into social isolation. A wise, caring pastor, able to talk to family and friends, can help everyone find ways to prevent this in providing spiritual support and positive pastoral care.

RELATIONSHIP WITH THE ENVIRONMENT

Opportunities to connect with the environment are essential for wholeness and spiritual health. This is so for the person with Alzheimer's disease, as I have written elsewhere in this book, and it is of equal importance to the care giver. God, the Creator, is revealed in creation. As indicated above, the spiritual yearning of a grieving care giver finds some fulfilment in the natural environment of the outdoors, especially where there is quiet and beauty. In spiritual yearning a person is often intensely aware of each small leaf, each bird's song, each tiny flower in roadside weeds, the lowing of beasts, the song of birds, the play of shadow and sunlight. All are cause for wonder and inner connectedness to the created world. All can help the healthy release of tears.

Other care givers will seek release in a cultural environment, finding spiritual renewal and refreshment in a choral or orchestral concert, a quilt exhibition or in the art gallery where paintings delight and inspire and sculpture can be touched and marvelled at.

I followed an intensive lecture tour of the UK by renewing my spirit among the primroses and violets, the tiny villages – and always the sea – of the North Devon countryside. On my way home, briefly visiting Florence and Rome, I stood in front of Michaelangelo's unutterably magnificent David and before the bronze doors of the baptistry. I felt tears of deep joy and thankfulness for the wonder of God's gifts of human creativity so perfectly manifest in these works. I knew that what I experienced was spiritual joy and wonder and that my tears were part of my tired spirit's renewal and communion with the Divine Spirit drawing me ever closer to my true self in love with the God-self, at one with the meaning and purpose of the universe.

Meaning and purpose

We all need a strong sense of knowing that life has meaning and purpose.

What is the meaning of life? That is the ultimate question. In the end each must answer from head and heart, and all alone. The meaning is found in the lived life. Not all at once but slowly, until we answer broken and despairingly with Shakespeare's Macbeth, 'a tale told by an idiot, full of sound and fury, signifying nothing', or in hands stretched to grasp the proffered fingers of God, as in Michelangelo's Sistine Chapel painting, *God creates Adam.* The difference is discovered in the grace of trusting – trusting the mystery that the nurtured spirit recognises as love, the goodwill of the Creator towards that which was made for love – the love of God.

Some of the most valuable work of the presbyter and parish family could be a gift of time and quiet for the care giver so that his or her innate creativity has opportunity for expression. Then there can be space to experience in art and literature, in solitude and silence, nobility of thought and form, and to ponder the naturally true and beautiful, to love and be loved in return and, in his or her religious belief and rituals and in the company perhaps of a spiritual guide, to explore the meaning of undeserved suffering.

This is spiritual work. A good pastor–presbyter, willing to be a spiritual companion in these circumstances, is able to empower the care giver towards wholeness from out of his or her own shared faith journey, his or her astute and scholarly knowledge of scripture. The tradition of the *anamchara* – 'the soul friend' – was established very early in the life of the Christian Church. St Brigit of the Christian Celtic tradition is reported as once saying that a person without a soul friend was like a body without a head. I know that in the reformed church culture there is a traditional resistance to anyone standing between the believer and God, but even this is being reviewed.

Particular areas of spiritual and emotional concern may arise for care givers as people with a primary dementia and their families face the

The main focus of communication should be on building relationships rather than seeking information. Asking questions can only further distance care giver and the person being cared for. God may seem to be very remote and unmoved. A pastoral presence which is caring and consistent, and able to share God's assurance of everlasting love in many and varied ways, can help to dispel the deep painful feelings of exile and alienation.

Commitment

Questions of commitment are bound to arise for every care giver. Spouses may worry about the commitment of loving 'for better for worse, in sickness and in health' when they perceive their partner as seemingly no longer the person to whom the commitment was originally made.

Many will be helped by an opportunity to share commitment concerns with a trusted pastor who would, of course, be foolish to rush in with 'answers'. What is required is empathetic paying attention and listening. The human heart and spirit are often capable of enormous and noble sacrifice and love. One care giver of his severely impaired wife, now in professional care, visited her every day to hold her hand, stroke her hair and face and in every way assure her of his continued loving. One day he said to me from his heart, 'I have loved her since I first set my eyes on her at the Sunday school picnic and I love her still. This is where I want to be – here beside her.' I am constantly humbled by the normalising power of such love.

In his keynote address to the Uniting Church is Australia's national conference on aged care, Dr Elbert Coles told of his experience in caring for his wife. An active parish minister, he decided early in his care giver role that his work could make it possible to keep her beside him. She stayed with him in the stream of life, stimulated by all kinds of sights and experience for seventeen years. Virginia never became violent, anxious, sad – or, as so many, like a silent, sitting hen. There were problems, though.

> We'd go to conferences where there would be two or three thousand people and you know what happens when sessions are over. Can you realise how quickly two people could get lynched if they held up a whole big facility just for them. So we found out those little hidden places around convention centres – the rest rooms that are off the bars and other places where Methodist ministers frequently gather, off the rooftop restaurants and all that. You know, people in our country have done a good business out of writing books on bed and breakfast establishments. I'm thinking of

writing a book on *Bathrooms Across America* – kinds that can best be used by spouses in our situation.

In Limon, Colorado they went into a men's room and as they were about to leave a man came in and got very excited.

> He…cursed and said, 'What's this so-and-so woman doing in this men's room? Can't you tell this is a men's room?' So I kind of thought, well, Elbert, you are a Methodist minister; you ought to think of something kind and helpful to say. Maybe you ought to think of something religious that you could say that would help this man. So I looked at him and I said, 'Oh, go to hell!' Virginia took my arm and we walked out. I don't know what she thought about it but I sure wasn't sure whether we'd get shot in the back or not. But, you know, we had a sense of feeling all right about it all.

His story is about brave, loving commitment. It illustrates how very important the care giver's attitude is in determining the quality of life for both the disabled person and the care giver. Openness is a very positive stance for the care giver to take. There is no shame in dementia and, the more open and honest care givers can be, the more understanding, kindness and informed support they are likely to receive. Brain failure, in the form of a dementia illness, is part of being human – as unfortunate a part of being human as are heart failure, hearing failure, kidney failure, and so on. But the experience is still human. Those who occupy that aspect of our human condition are not to be put aside or shunned.

Some care givers may want to raise questions of fidelity in a relationship where one partner may deteriorate so that he or she seems no longer to be the person to whom the commitment was made. Is 'for better or for worse, in sickness and in health' still binding? There is no easy answer to such a question.

The experience of care-giving may be faith-growing or faith-busting. There are some life circumstances that cannot be fixed. In this situation the role of the counsellor and the role of the spiritual guide are quite different. The pastor must decide which mantle he or she will claim. The counsellor may work with the care giver so that the question is resolved in such a way that allows the care giver to find a solution which is acceptable to him or her and which will allow him or her to live comfortably and without inner conflict in the particular circumstance.

The spiritual guide or companion will help the care-giver to find meaning and purpose in his or her undeserved suffering and deprivation and allow eventual acceptance without inner conflict of his or her life situation. If meaning and purpose can be found the grief and deprivation, although still painful, will not be destructive but ennobling. In the end it is important for the care giver's spiritual health to preserve his or her integrity.

Care givers generally struggle alone with questions of sexuality in dementia. It is my experience that it often remains the unspoken factor in discussion about transferring care to professionals. Recently I returned to the vastly different maternity hospital where my children were born. I marvelled at the double bed in each birthing room and sadly reflected on the absence of double beds in care homes for old people.

Although he did not specifically say so, my intuitive guess is that the question of sexuality was at the root of a request I received from a gentleman wanting small flat-like accommodation in which he and his wife with Alzheimer's disease could receive all the security and care services (meals, laundry, and so on) of the usual care home. He desired to live with his wife in a facility which allowed them the privacy of their own space and bedroom but relieved him of many of the burdens of caring in their own home, which he was finding beyond his capabilities. At the time I could not help him but subsequently I attended the opening of a new building for the Christchurch Methodist Mission; it could have provided this much-needed, humanised care environment.

Loss and death

The normal response to loss is grief, and care givers will grieve for the losses that Alzheimer's disease has brought and will continue to bring. The normal reactions to grief will most likely include denial, anger, bargaining, depression and, at last, acceptance. These are the classic elements of grief. They may not be experienced by every care giver in this order. Some people may not experience every stage. Some, if not care-fully supported, may get stuck at any stage. Many people simply do not understand that these states are normal. Anger and depression in grief are often difficult for friends and family to bear.

When Elbert Coles observed that people in his parish were beginning to avoid his wife in early-stage Alzheimer's disease he gathered the church elders, told them the full story and asked that the facts be quietly given out at appropriate times and places. He did not know it at the time, but a trained nurse undertook to visit each parish group and committee to provide a brief informal talk about Alzheimer's disease. Members were invited to ask questions and were told how best to communicate with Virginia and how to include her for as long as possible in the parish fellowship.

People enquired of Dr Coles how they could best support him. Two or three of Virginia's closest friends arrived each Monday and helped her to dress ready to go out with them for lunch. Because of their initiative he had almost all of his day off for his own needs and recreation. This continued until Virginia could no longer cope with the outing. Then the women stayed with her at home, always taking time and thoughtfulness to make it a pleasant day. Now that was a truly wonderful commitment to loving friendship.

Some people, who worried that Virginia's disease might be contagious, once they were empowered with knowledge, became among the most supportive. In this way losses for Dr Coles were minimised. He did not have to give up his work and known companions at the same time as slowly losing his loved mate's full participation in his life.

My own conviction is that as more and more people become aware of dementia illness there will be more people wanting to give assistance where it is needed most.

On transfer to professional care

For those caring for a loved person with a dementia illness the trauma of handing that care over to professional strangers is almost inevitable. However, no one person can provide the supervision and care which the latter stages of the disease demand. No matter how objective, wise, rational and reasonable the decision may be, the move will none the less be experienced as a severe displacement.

First, there is a complete change of status. The person with Alzheimer's disease will feel the loss but will not be able to understand why he or she feels so sad. The care giver will face loss, guilt, loneliness and endless inner questions which find their source not in the head but in the heart. It is a time when the church family, educated to the stresses and strains – as well as to the joy and loving of care-giving – can encourage and affirm the care giver. The presbyter can provide a useful affirming ministry by attending to four needs:

1. prayer

2. education for the care giver, especially in a visiting mode

3.   provision of a ritual to help the care giver hand over the responsibility of total physical care to others and to find new ways of demonstrating love

4.   encouragement for the care giver to reintegrate into the full life of the church family in the community.

PRAYER

Time spent on one's knees, holding needy people before God, is probably the presbyter's most important pastoral task. We can never do enough of it. Some parishes have organised prayer groups which pray especially for people with brain damage.

EDUCATION IN EFFECTIVE VISITING MODE

Try to imagine what it must be like to be a woman who had been married to someone for fifty years or more, living in the closest intimacy. Now you have to visit your spouse in the often-crowded lounge of a rest home for people with a primary dementia illness. You will be fortunate to find a seat to sit beside your loved one. He does not recognise you. You want to hug him but you cannot be sure how he may react. You are uneasy and self-conscious because of all the other residents in the lounge. Some of them shout or whine the same few words over and over. Some appear to be asleep, and all look lost, like refugees from another time and space. You have no privacy at all. Tears prick your eyes painfully. But you do not cry, not yet. You are aware of the other visitors. Most of them are as anxious and as uncomfortable as you are. Will you continue to stand before your husband's chair? You are too self-conscious to kneel; besides, you know you would not be able to get up again without help.

The experience is extremely painful for you. You tentatively touch your man and say his name. There is no response. He seems unaware of your presence, this man you love, this man who was once your young lover, husband, father of your children, companion of your days, is no more... His reality is not your reality and you cannot open the door into his place of forgetfulness. The worst of all is not being able to relate to each other. Does he know that you brought him to this place? Can he feel that you did not want to? Does he know how hard and long you tried to keep him at home with you? Can you tell him about the cold, empty space in your bed and the bitter-sweet joy of discovering the first rose flowering in his rose garden this morning – the one he bought with his overtime money when the first grandchild was born? You see in your mind his questioning grin when he showed it to you. You remember the mixture of exasperation and joy – that money was to have bought him a new pair of shoes for the baby's baptism. Now, although he sits there before you, you cannot say, 'Remember when…?' You want to put your head on his shoulder and cry your heart out but you have learned he needs your comforting and has none for you. And anyway, you know that for those who love, the heart can never be cried out.

You begin to wonder why you come to visit at all. Does your coming help him? Just one response would be enough – a smile, your name. But there is nothing. You turn to go and the hours until your next visit will be heavy with apprehension mixed with longing and hope.

Sadly, this is the daily experience of many care givers when they transfer their caring to professionals. As the baby boom generation enters the 60-plus years there will be many more care givers in this situation. An informed faith community, care home staff, pastor or presbyter can do much to make this situation more bearable. A presbyter could provide leadership to train others to help older people with a loved memory-impaired and confused person in residential care to learn how to visit creatively so that both the care giver and the person being cared for receive benefit. The answer is to tap into the feelings of the disabled person. This is especially helpful for those with an Alzheimer's disease type of dementia.

I developed a visiting mode when my mother was in care and have used it successfully in my pastoral work since then. The previous chapter explains this mode. If someone in the faith community – or indeed in the wider community – can learn to teach this mode to care givers who are new to visiting, it would improve the quality of life not only for them but for the disabled person as well.

Elsewhere in this book (Chapter 2) I have provided information about the communication deficits and Appendix 9 reproduces a pamphlet which is now used in several countries to assist families in visiting people with dementia.

Meaning is known both in the head and the heart. It is both rational and affective. We have largely lost the symbols of transcendence in Western culture. With them we have lost the clues which could have assisted us to answer questions pertaining to old age and loss, even the devastating losses of dementia illnesses. Despite the progress of our century we remain human, subject to pain and suffering, loss and death. Unlike our forebears we no longer have the private and community rituals and symbols to help us make sense of this part of life. Many try to do so in their heads and most find the answers seldom satisfy the heart.

It is time to reclaim our lost symbols or invent new ones. My Cornish and Irish Celtic Christian forebears referred the whole of life to a meaning and purpose which, although transcendent and 'beyond', guided them in carrying out tasks as humble and routine as the planting of the potatoes on such and such a saint's feast day. If my great-great-grandmother lost her thimble she got on with her life and let St Anthony find it for her. Usually he did! Wives committed the little fishing boats to the protection of a power greater than themselves and waited for the catch and their men with a measure of confidence. Many of us, especially women, are inventing new symbols to explain the unexplainable moments of life, especially its routine of moving on.

The most valuable asset a family care giver has for more satisfying visiting is knowledge of the loved one's life over a long period. If this can be utilised to cue or trigger the remote memory, care giver and person being cared for may communicate in the present by way of the past. With experience and confidence the care giver can also learn to affirm and accept all feelings, knowing that what the loved one is feeling is likely to be an indication of his or her present reality.

For a number of years now I have been providing teaching sessions for care givers who have reached this stage of the journey with dementia. Care givers are empowered to help improve the quality of life for themselves and their loved one when even a small measure of relationship is restored. One of my pet hobby-horses is that we should cease doing so much for our able 60 to 70 year olds and provide empowerment skills so that they are able to minister to those of 70 and 80-plus years. Most of us are healthier and happier when we know we are being really useful. Such young old people could have a very worthwhile ministry teaching their old (that is, 70-plus) friends how to visit their loved ones creatively.

MARKING THE TRANSITION

The twentieth century has brought significant gains in the length of human life. The most rapidly growing population group in the last years of the century is that of the 100 years plus group. This gain in human longevity is the fruit of medical and technological progress.

This phenomenon happens to coincide with a widespread spiritual malaise, experienced especially by older people as a sense of emptiness and meaninglessness. Frankl (1963) observes that, as the struggle for human survival has brought results, human beings are confronted with a new question: 'Survival for what?' (Kimble 1990). It seems that although most people on the planet today, at least in the Western culture, have the means to live they have lost a meaning to live for. The decline in respect of the spiritual dimension of living and the failure to provide for it in our lives has produced a crisis in our old age – the crisis of meaning.

For this reason I was particularly happy when I received a request in 1995 for some advice and possibly resources for a special ceremony. Bronwyn Lane, an Alzheimer's Society fieldworker, and Richard Waugh, a Methodist presbyter, had perceived a need for a ritual for care givers who had recently transferred a loved one to professional caring in a hospital or nursing home. As it happened I was at that time preparing a service for a similar purpose so I made a few suggestions about resources. Eventually they held their ceremony and sent me a copy, which is reproduced below. Any parish, perhaps working with the local Alzheimer's Society, could provide such a service. It would be a most relevant mission to their community. This ceremony is deeply appreciated by people who are not religious as well as regular church attenders.

A ceremony to mark the transfer of care of a family member

Prepared by Bronwyn Lane, ADARDS South Auckland and Rev. Richard Waugh, Trinity Methodist Church, Pakuranga, Auckland and used here with their kind permission.

> *Chairs are set out in a U shape. There is a low table in the centre with paper and marking pens on it and copies of music to be used. Lectern and flowers are at the front. There is a whiteboard beside the lectern with a large decorated circle outline on it. Each group is welcomed at the door as they arrive and each care giver given a corsage. The celebrants introduce themselves.*

Statement of occasion

Leader: You have been invited here today because in the past few months you have decided that the time has come to transfer your loved one with dementia to permanent rest home or hospital care. This ceremony provides an opportunity to formally acknowledge this

gaps but some relief too. And there will be new tasks and opportunities that you will be picking up, some easy, some difficult.

(*While speaking, place the following items on the low table in centre of the room: knife, fork and plate, set of keys, slippers, sheet, cheque book and £10 note.*)

We invited you to bring some item that is significant for you, something that relates to aspects of the caring task you have done or that may trigger thoughts about new tasks for you. I've added a few items that may stir more thoughts. I invite you now to share with people here the significance of your item or of any of the others here on the table. Share with us what you are giving away, the new tasks you are picking up. Nothing will be too trivial. Everyone here will understand.

(*Be prepared for a long pause, possibly prepare one member of the group or helpers to make an opening comment.*)

Comments from the group:

Leader: A new task that you face is visiting your family member in the new setting. Your bond with that person remains, but the relationship has changed and the caring task is different. One of the first difficulties that a lot of care givers face is the question, 'Will you take me home?' This poem may help you to deal with some of your feelings about it and to look at what you can do. (*Pause*)

Will you take me home?
I cannot take you home.
But I can comfort you when the floor shimmers like a sunlit lake.
I can wait while you layer, like memories, tissue precisely on tissue.
And remember for you, who you are and what you have done.
I can give you order and refuge in the strange land you inhabit now.
I can love you as you are...
But my hand cannot remould such a fragile piece as you.
I wish...but I cannot take you home. (Mandlen 1985)

Scripture and comment:

Leader: Here are some selected bible readings which give hope for our living. They are chosen especially for you as you rebuild your own lives and consider new tasks.

Psalm 88:12 (*Living Bible*)

Romans 8:35, 37–39 (*Good News Bible*)

Isaiah 40:28–31 (*Good News Bible*)

(*Set an eagle sculpture or symbol on the table among other symbols*)

Leader: The biblical image of the eagle is a symbol of strength and long life, a sign of blessing. The eagle is also seen as an image of God, carrying us, holding us up, protecting us like a young one is protected in the nest and helping us to soar. Picture yourself as the young eagle, helpless, needing to be fed, learning to fly. See how the parent eagle holds you up, encourages you, protects you. Then imagine yourself as an adult eagle with strong wings flying in the sky. Where do you get the strength to go on when you have used up all your own strength? Where do you turn for patience when you have run out of patience, when you have been more patient for more years than anyone should be asked to be, and the end is nowhere in sight?

I believe that God gives us strength and patience and hope, renewing our spiritual resources when they run dry. (Based on the words of Rabbi Harold Kushner 1988)

Let us all stand and together read the prayer for strength printed in your order of service.

Prayer:

All: **God of strength, who calls forth eagles to bend wings in adoration, who sends forth eagles to wing wide in praise, I am in need of your strength.**
I am weary, tired, unable to soar in my sky of life. Carry me on your loving wings. Renew my strength. Give me the energy for the going and create in me an openness to future flying.
Great God of eagles' hearts, I want to trust that you will bear me up, that you will support me. I look to you to renew my strength just as surely as eagles' wings are wide in the sky. Amen

Leader: Now, as we remain standing, I invite you to close your eyes, lift up your head and receive the strength of God. Let it flow through you.

(*Allow time for silence*)

Closing prayer:

Loving God, we give you thanks for this gathering today, for the care of others, for the support of family and friends. Thank you for the comfort and encouragement of this ceremony and for the strength you give us to manage the changes ahead. We ask now for your blessing on our families and especially on our loved ones now in care.

Let us pray together the Lord's Prayer.

(*Use the traditional version*)

Hymn: 'One More Step Along the World I Go'
(*Introduced by*)

Leader: Our closing song today talks about hope for the future. The music is available for anyone for whom it may be unfamiliar.

Blessing:

Leader: Go in faith and live a life that is pleasing to God.
            May faith, hope and love go with you. Amen.

(*Make announcements as needed about the invitation to remain to share a cup of tea or coffee, food and conversation together and handouts such as 'Visiting the Person with Dementia', and so on*)

One would not have to be part of this ceremony to feel the power of the use made of symbols. People have been involved at a very deep level. It has the great merit that because it is a small, intimate event it can be provided more frequently than the larger celebration described below. It could therefore be offered quite soon after any one transfer of care has taken place. It is also acceptable to non church-goers.

We turn now to a liturgy I prepared for a larger ecumenical occasion to serve a similar purpose to the foregoing. This one is less intimate and personal, placing the care givers' needs into the company of God's people. It reminds us that there is a sense in which the pain of one member of the body becomes the shared pain of all.

Both services are healing and seriously received by care givers and their families. The best liturgies are those prepared for a particular people and context.

Liturgy for journeying on

We acknowledge the past, we grieve and we move on.

This is a service of consolation and hope for those who have recently made the hard decision to transfer the care of one they love to permanent rest home or hospital. The liturgy is prepared especially for care givers of people with Alzheimer's disease or other related dementia. It is envisaged that it would take place in the context of the worshipping community in a parish or ecumenical setting.

Introduction, welcome and notices:

Greetings:

Leader: The Lord be with you

People: And also with you.

Statement of intention:

Leader: We have come together in the presence of God to acknowledge the hard journey of those among us who find that loving now means transferring the care of one they love to residential rest home or hospital care. We have come to declare God's faithfulness and to reach out in practical love and concern to all those who must bear one of the most painful losses of old age.

People: Eternal God, you are our dwelling place and underneath are your everlasting arms.

Hymn: 'Praise to the Lord, the Almighty, the King of creation'

Remembering who we are:

Leader: Let us now remember who we are.

People: We are people called to do justice, love kindness and to walk humbly with our God.

Leader: Now and always we are the sons and daughters of the Living God.

People: Amen. We are the people of God and into our hearts has been given that love which is for the healing of the nations. The power of Christ is in us.

Leader: While life can be hard we will not despair for we claim the grace of God towards us.

People: **Amen. In the Holy Spirit we celebrate our energy and strength to hold fast, our power to heal, and our calling to walk humbly with God.**

Leader: Some among us grieve. Life has not turned out for them and their loved one – spouse, parent or friend – as the start of the journey seemed to promise. Now there is a new kind of separation and confusion and sometimes a frightening mix of emotions which is part of transition. Now is the trembling beginning of a new journey.

Response liturgy:

Leader: All of life is a journey on many different roads.

People: **Guard us, O Lord, as the apple of your eye.**
Shelter us under the shadow of your wings.

Leader: Sometimes the way is easy.
Sunlight falls on our faces and the wind is at our backs.

People: **Guard us, O Lord, as the apple of your eye.**
Shelter us under the shadow of your wings.

Leader: There is also a hard and lonely way through steep and narrow tracks of sorrow and fear in dark places.

People: **Guard us, O Lord, as the apple of your eye.**
Shelter us under the shadow of your wings.

Leader: Whatever the journey, we are not alone. God is with us.

Hymn: 'Where the road runs out and the signposts end' or 'One more step along the road we go'

The Reading of the Word:

> Hebrew Scriptures: Isaiah 43:1–3
>
> The Letters: Romans 8:35, 37–39
>
> The Gospel: John 1:1–5, 14

Contemporary witness: homily or reflection

(*My theme was from John 1:15. Light: Life, Insight, Power. I used a solar-powered pocket calculator as an illustration of light as power.*)

Choir: anthem or solo

Turning to the Light for the Way Ahead:

Leader: This poem is for those on a new journey of caring. Let it help you to value your new way of caring – a caring only you can give.

First Reader:

            Will you take me home?

Second Reader:

            I cannot take you home
            But I can comfort you when the floor shimmers like a sunlit lake.
            I can wait while you layer, like memories, tissue precisely on tissue,
            And remember for you, who you are, and what you have done.
            I can give you order and refuge in the strange land you inhabit now.
            I can love you as you are...
            But my hand cannot remould such a fragile piece as you.
            I wish...but I cannot take you home. (Mandlen 1985)

Lighting of candle:

(*The candle should be large and beautiful and surrounded by low, small flowers and sprigs of rosemary for remembrance.*)

Leader: This candle is a symbol of Christ who said, 'I am the Light of the World.'

(*The candle is lit and those beginning their new journey are invited to come near to it.*)

Leader: This candle is a sign of light for your journey; light for the illumination of your mind, light for your life and growing, light which is power for costly loving, freely given.

            Feel the warmth of the flame. It is a sign of the warmth of God's love for you and our love for you. This love will be with you on your new journey. This love will enfold your special loved one.

            The power of the Holy Spirit who always moves ahead of you, grant you strength for your way, encouragement for those who journey with you, and that compassion for all who suffer which will draw you into the compassionate heart of Jesus, which is our healing. Amen.

(If desired, a small candle could be lit from the large candle and given to each person.)

Hymn of Commissioning: 'I am the Light of the World'

Prayer of Intercession:
(This prayer should especially include all care givers and all who suffer severe memory impairment and failing abilities.)

The Lord's Prayer: (This would be the traditional version.)

Hymn of Commitment: 'He came singing love' (or another of choice)

Blessing and Dismissal:
Leader:

> God be your comfort and strength,
> God be your hope and support;
> God be in you, above you, under you and around you.
> And the blessing of God, Creator, Redeemer and Giver
> of life remain with you now and always. Amen.

All: **Amen. (*sung*)**

Leader: Go into the world in peace.

All: **Amen. We go in the name of Christ.**

Acknowledgement:
Some of the above service was inspired by Dorothy McRae-McMahon's *Echoes for our Journey – Liturgies of the People*, published by the Joint Board of Christian Education, Melbourne, 1993 and is used with permission.

See also the suggested service for blessing a studio unit or sheltered housing flat given in Appendix 7.

Ministering to professional care givers

I have a dream...

I long to see private hospital and care home management making intentional provision for the pastoral care not only of their residents but also for staff. Those who care for people with dementia, especially those well advanced into the disease, do a magnificent task for the community for very little recognition in terms of status or financial reward. Most care givers, even registered nurses, admit to knowing very little about dementia illness when they first begin working with older people who are significantly cognitively impaired. Being with people whose reality is not your own can be very stressful.

For the pastor to be invited (or for him or her to ask for an invitation) to a staff morning coffee or afternoon tea break, especially after a number of deaths in the home or ward, can provide an opportunity to get to know staff on an informal basis. If confidence and mutual trust are present genuine caring and sharing may take place.

In my work I have found that professional care givers close to the resident often grieve profoundly when that person dies. It is natural. After all, a care giver may have been involved with the now-dead resident over a number of years. Care givers sometimes grieve also as they observe the deterioration of those around them. Genuine affection is often present. Accompanying people in a slow, insidious dying is a difficult, even courageous task. Being present involves recognition of what it means to be human and therefore mortal, of acknowledging the pain of being involved with the loss of abilities, insight and personality, and intentionally addressing the spiritual needs of those affected by the disease and those who accompany them in the journey.

A short memorial service held in the context of the regular or occasional service of worship, if there is one, can give expression to thankfulness for all that a disabled elder has done to enrich the lives of others just by 'being'. It can close a life for the care givers or others in the institution and grant them permission to share grief and memories, tears and faith.

A word about children

Generally, younger children accept forgetfulness and confusion. They seem to find it easier to relate to old people than do the other adults in a family. They are able to do what few adults achieve. They accept the old, confused person as he or she is in the present moment. Often both child and old person enjoy each other exceedingly well. They seem to understand and accept each other's wisdom.

My grandson, David, was six years old at the time of what proved to be my mother's last Christmas with us in the busy and crowded lounge where family, friends and neighbours were enjoying a light-hearted affair with mammon as gifts and food were exchanged and drinks were the order of the late morning. I can still see a neat, grey head and a small shining blond one close together. Little David's hand was tucked into his great-grandmother's. There was much noise but reading mother's lips I knew that she was asking over and over 'Whose birthday is it? Whose birthday is it?' David's back was towards me so I do not know how many times he answered or even if he had answered her before. But in a lull of conversation everyone heard his clear, sweet voice answer: 'It's Jesus' birthday, Nana. Jesus' birthday.'

'That's lovely, dear,' said mother in a 'settled' kind of voice. David turned so that I knew they smiled at each other.

At that moment the Christ-mass truly entered our hearts. These two, the oldest and youngest, had re-mind-ed and re-member-ed us all into family, into community, and bonded us together within that tender mystery whose name is 'God with us' (Emmanuel). Great truths enter our hearts out of such simplicity.

Pastors can help younger parent care givers understand that children will not suffer from having a confused memory-impaired old grandparent loved and warmly included in the home with them. Rather, there is considerable opportunity for blessing. Where love is demonstrated in the home every day, children are capable of living unharmed through a good deal of stress and tension which may be present around them but not aimed at them. Children, even little children, are capable of understanding and forgiving in their own way the tiredness and small weaknesses of the adults in their lives.

There seems to be an idea abroad in contemporary society that it is somehow damaging to expose our children to intergenerational experiences as if the very young and the very old were not good for each other. What nonsense! If our children are to inherit all that is best in their own Church and family, it must be shared and caught in hearts and minds while they are still children. And who can they catch the faith and cultural treasures from other than from those who have already lived a long life.

Summary

This chapter has attempted to offer practical guidelines for nurturing and maintaining the spiritual well-being of the person who cares at home for a family member with dementia. It does not attempt to cover other important aspects of caring for the care giver.

It identifies burdens that the care giver is likely to face. They are:

- social isolation
- grief
- lack of time for self, family and friends
- the heavy physical labour of care-giving (most care givers are 70-plus years of age)
- loss of hobbies and pursuit of new interests
- fulfilment of long-term retirement goals.

For some care givers there will be disruption and lost promotion opportunities. Almost all will experience continuing grief and guilt.

The affective context of care givers is examined with reference to the research of Anne Opie of Victoria University (1991). We have identified the spiritual needs of care givers as being associated with:

- maintaining a right relationship with God – the transcendent and immanent Other – oneself, others and the environment
- maintaining a sense of identity
- maintaining a strong sense that life has personal meaning and purpose even in the undeserved and difficult circumstances of caring for a loved person with dementia.

Suggestions for meeting these needs are discussed.

7

A Statement of Hope
The Field in Anathoth

And now faith, hope, and love abide, these three; but the greatest of these is love. (I Cor 13:13)

Now I end as I began, with a story. It is a kind of universal story, for we find versions of it in almost every culture and race.

Once there was an old man who lived with his son and daughter-in-law and their young son. They lived on a fine farm and in a beautiful house. The old man's great-grandfather had developed the land wisely. And they lived well in the lovely old house the old man's father had built for his young bride. It was far from the little cottage the old man's great-grandfather had built as quickly as possible because the land cried out for caring and the company of seeds and animals. Now the young man and his family enjoyed both and had been able to acquire some fine paintings, good furniture, precious carpets and other valuable possessions. They loved their house and the beautiful garden and well-tended farm.

Indeed, they loved that house so much that it irritated them that, as the old man grew more forgetful, feeble and confused, he was often messy and clumsy. One evening a fine china dinner plate was broken as he attempted to help his daughter-in-law clear the dinner table.

'That's it!' said the young man to his wife later that night. 'That's it! He'll have to eat his meals on the back porch. I'll make a couple of rough wooden bowls. I won't eat at the table with him again. Oh yes, yes, I know he's old but I won't have the mess. Besides, his spills will spoil the polished surface of the tabletop. And our china is expensive.'

And so the bowls were made and the old man sat exiled and lonely, stripped of the last remnants of his dignity, without cloth or napkin, at an old battered table in the porch.

Only the little boy missed him in the warm dining-room. He did not understand why his grandfather now ate alone in the porch. But he did notice the wooden bowls. One day his father found him busy with wood, hammer and chisel.

'What are you making, son?' asked the father.

'I'm making a bowl for you, Daddy, for when you're old and like Grandpa,' answered the child.

That evening the old man took his place with the family around the polished table, no longer an exile.

As I think of those who suffer dementia and those who care for them in an environment in which even the compassion of good people is more and more selective, I find hope and meaning in the biblical story of the ancient Hebrews' experience of exile in the strange world of ancient Babylon to which they were taken after the fall of their sacred city, Jerusalem. Like the exiled Hebrews, those suffering dementia have no choice about being separated from the mainstream of life. Care givers have little choice either and may wonder why their exile is so hard and long. Hope abides in remembering that exile is only a portion of the Hebrews' story. In the course of time an exiled nation came home.

But for now, while the Hebrews, trapped in besieged Jerusalem, lamented the forced abandonment of their homes and the decay of their lands made valueless because no one was there to care for them, and even as the Babylonian siege engines breached the walls of the city, the prophet Jeremiah negotiated to buy a field at Anathoth (see Jeremiah 32:1–44) at a *fair market price*. It was an act of economic lunacy. Even his own prediction was that Babylon would overcome them and take them into captivity and exile.

Buying that field was, on the face of it, absolutely crazy and we can be sure that many people told him that. No doubt Jeremiah felt foolish. So why did this most practical man do it? It all depends from which premise you start. Jeremiah's experience of God convinced him that God's purposes for his people are always for good and blessing. Jeremiah's purchase of the field in Anathoth was actually a sound and practical investment in what he believed would be a better future. It was also a profound declaration that nothing, no matter how valueless, is of no worth in the eyes of God.

God's people might feel totally deserted in the collapse of their nation but God had not forgotten them. There would be another and better time. Above all, when Jeremiah bought that field in Anathoth he made concrete a tangible statement of hope. All deliberate acts of hope are an invitation to ridicule because they are seen as foolishly out of touch with visible reality; they are counter-culture. However, I believe that our acts of hope are the reality which is being made but which is not yet clearly seen. Hope is our committed action connecting with God's action-in-the-world.

It is taking seriously that reality Benland (1988) spoke of before the Royal Commission on Social Policy in New Zealand: the 'something more, *taha wairua*' which, while it cannot be seen and measured, has such reality and importance that to ignore it imperils the fabric of our society and our very lives. Pragmatism (the belief that if something works it is right and true) is wearing thin for some in today's Church and society.

Even so, change comes very slowly and the experience of dementia for care givers and even their advocates usually comes at a stage of life which bears with it a sense of urgency. How much time do I have left to me to make any worthwhile difference? The thing about faithful loving in the circumstance of dementia illness is this: on the face of it, it makes no difference at all. No matter how much love is poured out, the condition gets no better; indeed it worsens.

In our heads we know that no amount of love can cure dementia. Love is defeated. Nevertheless, how many care givers' hearts continue to hope? How do we meet their pain or even the pain in our own hearts except by unconditional loving even when love appears to be defeated?

It is this kind of loving that empowers us to transcend defeat. It has a strange kind of honour that keeps human beings truly human – the divine spirit's greatest glory, according to St Irenaeus. In defeated love there is always a germ of new life. It is miracle. It is also a great suffering. And it is our hope.

Lionel (whose story I told in the previous chapter) understood this when he contemplated the man Jesus 'on that bloody cross'. That was a circumstance of defeated love too. But 'that bloody cross' is also the symbol of defeated love's power, in the person of the human man Jesus, to overcome the powers of chaos and darkness. It offers to all creation a new life of order and harmony in a community in which there are no exiles.

Suggested reading

The following are general books about Alzheimer's disease and related dementias.

Bailey, S. and Darling, J. (2001) *Tangles and Starbursts: Living with Dementia.* Alzheimer's Society – North Tyneside Branch.

Cheston, R. and Bender, M. (1999) *Understanding Dementia.* London: Jessica Kingsley Publishers.

Clayton, H., Graham, N. and Warner, S. (2002) *Dementia: Alzheimer's and Other Dementias.* London: Class Publishing.

Gidley, I. and Shears, R. (1988) *Alzheimer's: What it is and How to Cope.* London: Unwin Hyman.

Gilleard, C. (1984) *Living with Dementia.* London: Croom Helm.

Holden, U.F. (1990) *Dementia: Some Common Misunderstandings.* Bicester: Winslow (especially Chapter 6).

Jorm, A.F. (1987) *Understanding Senile Dementia.* London: Croom Helm.

Sacks, O. (1985) *The Man who Mistook his Wife for a Hat.* London: Duckworth.

Wattis, J. (1988) *Confusion in Old Age.* London: BMA (available through Alzheimer's Society, UK).

The following are selected for the use of care givers, family, presbyters and pastors.

Armstrong, L. and Reymbaut, E. (ed Chapman) (1996) *Getting the Message Across.* Stirling: University of Stirling.

Burton-Jones, J. (1992) *Caring for Care-givers.* London: Scripture Union.

Clark, G. (1993) *People Skills for Helpers.* Palmerston North: Dunmore.

Davis, R. (1989) *My Journey into Alzheimer's Disease.* Wheaton, IL: Tyndale (also Scripture Press 1993).

Froggatt, A. (1990) *Family Work with Elderly People.* London: Macmillan.

Goldsmith, M. (1996) *Hearing the Voice of People with Dementia.* London: Jessica Kingsley Publishers.

Hammond, G. and Mofitt, L. (2000) *Spiritual Care: Guidelines for Care Plans.* Leeds: Christian Council on Ageing and Faith in Elderly People.

Honel, R.W. (1988) *Journey with Grandpa – Our Family's Struggle with Alzheimer's Disease.* Baltimore: John Hopkins University Press.

Keunning, D. (1987) *Helping People Through Grief.* Minneapolis: Bethany House.

Killick, J. and Allan, K. (2001) *Communication and the Care of People with Dementia.* Buckingham: Open University Press.

Kitwood, T. and Bredin, K. (1992) *Person to Person – A Guide to the Care of Those with Failing Mental Powers.* Loughton: Gale Centre.

Kitwood, T. (1997) *Dementia Reconsidered.* Buckingham: Open University Press.

Kitwood, T. and Benson, S. (1995) *The New Culture of Dementia Care.* London: Hawker Publications.

Manning, D. (1990) *When Love Gets Tough – The Nursing Home Dilemma.* San Francisco: Harper.

Marshall, M. (1996) *I Can't Place This Place at All.* London: Venture Press.

Marshall, M. (ed) (1997) *State of the Art in Dementia Care.* London: Centre for Policy on Ageing.

Murphy, C. (1988) *Day to Day Spiritual Help When Someone You Love has Alzheimer's.* Philadelphia: Westminster.

Opie, A. (ed) (1991) *Caring Alone: Looking After the Elderly Confused at Home.* Wellington NZ: Daphne Brassell Associates.

Saunders, J. (2002) *Dementia: Pastoral Theology and Pastoral Care.* Cambridge: Grove Books.

The following selection is offered for church leaders and policy makers in any helping profession serving older people.

De Beauvoir, S. (1977) *Old Age.* London: Penguin.

Edwards, T.A. (ed) (1984) *Living the Apocalypse – Spiritual Resources for Social Compassion.* San Francisco: Harper.

Garland, J. (1991) *Making Residential Care Feel Like Home.* Bicester: Winslow.

Holden, U. (1987) *Looking at Confusion – A Handbook for Those Working with the Elderly.* Bicester: Winslow.

Marshall, M. (ed) (1990) *Working with Dementia: Guidelines for Professionals.* Birmingham: Venture Press.

Paul, S.S. and Paul, J.A. (1994) *Humanity Comes of Age – The New Context for Ministry with the Elderly.* Geneva: World Council of Churches.

Thomas, L.E. and Eisenhandler, S. (1994) *Ageing and the Religious Dimension.* London: Auburn.

The following may be useful for reading to children.

Fox, M. (1984) *Wilfrid Gordon McDonald Partridge.* Norwood, SA: Omnibus.

Guthrie, D. (1986) *Grampa Doesn't Know Me.* New York: Human Sciences Press.

The venue for worship

Some requirements

Here is a suggested list of requirements for a venue which is to be used for a worship service with people with Alzheimer's disease and their families, carers and friends.

The property

- The architecture must be recognisable as a church to assist people with memory cueing and orientation.
- Plenty of accessible off-street parking must be available.
- Wheelchair access is required.

The worship centre

- There must be accessible toilets nearby, clearly indicated by signs.
- Good, comfortable seating, preferably single chairs, must be provided; if pews have to be used they must be generously spaced.
- There must be a good musical instrument, preferably an organ, and a competent organist.
- There must be wide aisles for wheelchair access.
- A good sound system should be available.
- There needs to be a pleasant, convenient location for serving refreshments after the service.
- Warmth is important.
- Afternoon tea should be served after worship. This is an excellent opportunity for sharing and fellowship. Alzheimer's Society members and some church members may like to share the preparation and serving of tea.

Service of the word, prayer and praise

This order of worship is planned to meet the needs of older people with failing mental powers (Alzheimer's disease and related disorders) in a care home, hospital or day care setting. It could also be used in their own homes for those unable to attend their local church if holy communion is not appropriate. The service works best when family and friends are invited, along with representatives of the local congregation – they help with the responses and the singing and help make community.

Orientation and greetings:

Leader: Good afternoon everyone. It is good to be at church with you again. Today is (*name of day*). We are at (*name of care home*). You live here. Some people are visitors. I am (*own name*). I am the minister. I am leading our worship. (*Name of pianist*) is playing the piano. We are the church in this place. We have come together to hear God's word, to worship and to praise God. We have come together to encourage each other.

Call to worship:

Minister: God is here.

People: God is always here.

Minister: God is with us.

People: God is always with us.

All: Thanks be to God. Amen.

Hymn: All things bright and beautiful'

Prayers of Approach and Confession:

Leader: Spirit of God, come to help us and lead us to peace.

All: Amen.

Leader: Let us now come closer to God with sincerity of heart and fully assured that our Father God loves us. Let us confess our sins.

People: **Lord God, we have not always loved you; we have not always loved each other as you have loved us. We have not loved ourselves. Lord, we are truly sorry. Have mercy on us. Amen.**

                 (*A little silence*)

Absolution:

Leader: Dear people, in the name of Jesus Christ, I tell you, we are forgiven.

All: **Amen.**

The Peace:

(*Visitors are invited to move around and greet other visitors and to pass the Peace to the residents as well as to each other. It may be necessary to demonstrate this since it is better to approach people with dementia slowly from the front, take both hands, make eye contact and say:* 'The peace of Christ be with you'.)

Old Testament Reading:

Psalm 23. (*Invite the people to recite it with you. Many people with dementia will do this.*)

Hymn: 'What a Friend we have in Jesus'

Gospel reading: Matthew 19:13–15

Good News Sentences:

Leader: The little children wanted to be near Jesus. The disciples thought Jesus was too busy to be bothered with children. Jesus said: Let the little children come to me and do not stop them. Jesus wants everyone to be his friend. Jesus wants us because he loves us. Jesus loves you.

All: **Amen.**

Hymn: 'Abide with Me'

Pastoral prayer:

Leader: God, our Father, we love you and we want to love you more. You never forget us. We are your people. Help us to rest in your strength for you are the loving arms around all of your creation. Guard, guide and keep us and those we love as the apple of your eye. Use our weakness to make others strong. Keep your church in truth, keep our world in goodwill and bless each one of us.

We pray in Jesus' name. Amen

The Lord's Prayer: (traditional version)

Blessing:

Leader: The Lord bless you and keep you; the Lord make his face to shine on you and be gracious to you.

The Lord lift up the light of his countenance upon you and give you peace.

Amen.

Benediction:

Leader: The grace of our Lord Jesus Christ,
the love of God and the fellowship of the Holy Spirit
be with you always.
Amen.

A note for ministers:

Some have questioned the use of confession and absolution; the difficulty seems to be the degree to which people with failing mental powers can be responsible for their relationship with God. Ministers will have to answer that question for themselves. For myself the issue is that none of us can hear God's forgiveness often enough. That 'my people' are forgiven is the good news I bring to them each time we worship together.

A celebration of Holy Communion

An order prepared for people with Alzheimer's disease and related dementia, their families and friends, and also visitors and staff in a hospital or care home setting. The able support the disabled with the responses. (This liturgy can also used for a home communion).

Greetings and orientation:

Leader: Good morning everyone. I am very happy to be with you again. Today is (*name of day*). We are at (*name of place*). It is a (*windy? warm?*) day. I am (*own name*). I will lead our celebration. (*Name*) is playing the piano. We have come together to meet our Lord in the communion of his body and blood. We have come to worship God and to encourage each other with our love.

Preparation:

Leader: The Lord be with you.

People: And also with you.

Leader: God is here.

People: God is always here.

Leader: God is here with us.

People: God is always here with us. Amen.

Prayer of approach:

All: Almighty God, to whom all hearts are open, all desires known and from whom no secrets are hidden, cleanse the thoughts of our hearts by your Holy Spirit that we may truly love you and worthily praise your holy name; through Jesus Christ our Lord. Amen.

Hymn

Confession:

Leader: We have come together to hear God's word and to meet our Lord in the communion of his body and blood. Let us therefore seek God's grace that we may come in repentance and faith.

All: **Lord, we have not always loved you with all our heart; we have not always loved our neighbour as ourselves; we have not always loved one another as you have loved us. Have mercy on us.**

(*A short silence is kept.*)

Leader: God's mercy never ends. In the name of Jesus Christ you/we are forgiven.

People: **Thanks be to God.**

Ministry of the Word:

> Bible reading
>
> Gospel sentences

Hymn

Ministry of the Sacrament:

Leader: The peace of God be with you.

People: **And God's peace be with you.**

(*The people – visitors and staff – are then invited to take Christ's peace to each other, their own special loved resident and the special residents of other visitors.*)

Leader: Lift up your hearts.

People: **We lift them to the Lord.**

Leader: Let us give thanks to the Lord our God. Let us pray.

> Loving God, we praise you and thank you. Heaven and earth are full of your glory. You are always thinking about us. We are your people; you never forget us. In the life, death and resurrection of Jesus Christ you have shown us that nothing can destroy your love or separate us from you.

People: **Amen. Glory to the Father and to the Son and to the Holy Spirit; as it was in the beginning is now and ever shall be; world without end. Amen.**

Leader: We recall that on the night before he died Jesus was sharing a Passover meal with his disciples. He took bread and after giving thanks, broke it and gave it to this disciples saying, 'Take, eat, this is my body which is given for you. Do this in remembrance of me.' Then he took the cup after supper and said, 'This cup is the new covenant in my blood. Whenever you drink it, do this in remembrance of me.

Prayer to the Holy Spirit:

Leader: Come, Holy Spirit, that these gifts of bread and wine may be to us the bread of life and the cup of salvation. Bind us into one body, that we may grow into the fulness of Christ who is the head. Amen.

The Breaking of the Bread:

Leader: The bread which we break is a sharing in the body of Christ. The cup of blessing for which we give thanks is a sharing in the blood of Christ. Amen.

(A short silence)

Leader: Behold, the lamb of God who takes away the sin of the world.

The Communion:

Leader: Draw near in faith and take this holy sacrament in remembrance that Christ died for you and feed on him in your hearts with thanksgiving.

(The bread and wine of the communion is served with these words: [name] Christ's body, broken for you; [name] The blood of Christ, poured out for you.)

Prayer after Communion

Leader: Most loving, Holy Lord, creator and redeemer, with all our hearts we give you thanks for this foretaste of your glory.

People: Amen.

Leader: Let us pray:

People: Our Father, who art in heaven. Hallowed by thy name. Thy kingdom come, thy will be done on earth as it is in heaven. Give us this day our daily bread; and forgive us our trespasses as we forgive those who trespass against us. And lead us not into temptation but deliver us from evil. For thine is the kingdom, the power and the glory for ever and ever. Amen.

Blessing

Dismissal:

Leader: Go in peace.

People: Amen. We go in the name of Christ.

(Note: Serving may take some time. Do not hurry. It is good to have extra servers. Often Christian staff members will be delighted to be asked to serve their patients/residents in this way.)

An ecumenical service

This is a service I prepared for people with Alzheimer's disease, their care givers, families and friends. The service was widely publicised in the city because we hoped that people with very limited contact with older people with brain failure would come. It was also an opportunity for ordinary people to honour the work care givers do for the community and to demonstrate care and concern. Many people tell me that they have been deeply moved and energised by the 'outpouring of love' which they experience at these events.

The local Alzheimer's Society has always supported this service and taken part in its organisation. Its officers have been involved in leading the worship. When the Society recently invited me to act as their advisor in the spiritual dimension of care they accepted responsibility for sponsoring the ecumenical worship service. The Church, represented by myself, is responsible for content and leadership.

Leader:	'Loving kindness in the Land of Forgetfulness?'
People:	**Yes, for while life can be hard we are not defeated.**
Leader:	We come together to worship God and to affirm our faith.
People:	**Yes, in the face of all that seems against us, we own the grace of God towards us.**
Leader:	What can separate us from God's love? There is nothing in life or death than can separate us from God's love for us in Jesus Christ.

Welcome, greetings and orientation

Call to worship:

Leader:	God is here.
People:	**God is always here.**
Leader:	God is with us.
People:	**God is always with us.**
All:	**The Lord's name be praised. Amen.**

Prayer of approach and confession

Absolution

Hymn: 'What a friend we have in Jesus'

Scripture readings: Psalm 46:1–5, 7, 10–11; Luke 9: 12–17

Good News sentences

Distribution of Bread

Hymn: 'Jesus loves me'

Prayer of confidence

The Lord's Prayer (traditional version)

Hymn: 'All people that on earth do dwell' (3 verses)

Blessing and dismissal

(*This public service has been used to mark the beginning of Alzheimer's Disease Awareness Week.*)

(*Note on Good News Sentences: These expand the reading in no more than two or three very short one-thought sentences. The message I want people to hear from this particular scripture, 'Feeding the Five Thousand', is this: very little becomes much – a lot – when given to Jesus. In the hands of Jesus our little gift becomes much – it becomes a blessing for many. (That's all! That is enough!)*)

Occasionally a fellow clergyperson will say something like this: 'Well, Eileen, I understand why you want to keep it short and simple but have you thought about the care givers? An awful lot come and probably going to church is a rare experience for many of them. Don't you think you should preach something a little more solid for them? After all, they are there.'

My answer is that this ministry is about gently empowering profoundly handicapped people to walk with some sense of 'accompanying' and confidence into the Kingdom of Heaven. It is not about numbers in pews or feeding sheep who are well able to seek out their own pasture. This service is for 'resting in'. I hope care givers will experience that with us. They tell me they do and are often moved to tears by the responses of loved ones. An ecumenical worship service for people with Alzheimer's disease and their care givers should not be a poor, little and mean affair. The Church needs to bring out all its treasures: music, rich, old and noble words, vestments, colour, stained glass windows, gleaming candlesticks, incense, flowers and ritual for a glorious celebration in praise of God.

Regarding the distribution of bread, this ritual is symbolic of God's gracious love for his people and his provision for our needs, regardless of our usefulness in the world. It is a way for the Church to say with Christ: 'You are loved. You are God's precious children. God never forgets us. By God's grace the Church will not forget you either.'

Bread in a large basket with colourful paper napkins is placed on the communion table or altar. Representatives of the assembly take these small loaves to the congregation and give each person a piece of bread and a short blessing, 'God loves you', or 'Bless you'. Our experience is that people are very quiet and reverent. For some it is necessary to put the bread into their mouths.

Another way to say this is with perfumed oil (especially if linked to the story of Jesus' anointing in Mark 14:3–9). Instead of the bread baskets there could be small china or wooden trinket boxes or attractive little bowls, each containing a small wad of cotton wool soaked in perfumed oil. People distributing the perfumed oil could press a thumb into the cotton wool and trace the sign of the cross on each person's forehead or palm. They would offer a blessing as with the bread.

There are many other creative ways by which the Church can minister an effective worship ministry to people who can no longer remember. There is no doubt in the minds of those who assist with this ritual that people with dementia know that this is a special occasion.

Appendix 6

A Christmas service

This is an ecumenical service of carols and readings for people with Alzheimer's disease and related dementia, their care givers, families and friends.

This service was held in an inner city church on a Sunday afternoon early in December.

In the sanctuary we made a little live tableau of the manger, the Christ child and Mary his mother who was a little girl from my own congregation – Joseph should have been there, too, but unhappily he went down with measles. Mary was wonderful; she fed her baby, burped him, rocked him in her arms and just gazed at him in the straw. This beautiful tableau centred our people and kept their attention.

Other ministers working with people with Alzheimer's disease in parish or care home settings assisted with readings.

We served Christmas cake with tea in the church after the service. This had been donated by a major food manufacturer.

The service provided an opportunity for many older, active people to use their talents to serve others. The Salvation Army Veteran's Band provided incidental music and leadership for some of the carols. The Army's involvement in Christmas carols played from the back of a truck is a long-time New Zealand tradition and provided a strong cue for remote memories of the Christmas season and our Lord's birth. In the UK leading up to Christmas Salvation Army bands often play in town centres and residential neighbourhoods.

Remembering with joy and hope

Welcome, notices, orientation

Call to Worship

Leader: God is here.

People: God is always here.

Leader: God is with us.

Blessing of a sheltered housing or studio unit in a home for older people with failing mental powers

This liturgy is taken from A New Zealand Prayer Book. This is acknowledged with gratitude.

All units tend to open off a common room or hall in this type of accommodation. People are invited to bring their own furniture, favourite ornaments, pictures, and so on. In my view it is an excellent option for some confused elderly people transferring into institutional care from a private home.

A ceremony to mark the beginning of this life may be appropriate. Family and a few friends could be invited. The service is sometimes followed with the Eucharist if that is desired and always with a celebratory afternoon tea.

The order of service should be printed and copied attractively with the occupant's name, the clergyperson's name and it should record those who were invited to be present. I find that in the weeks following, the printed service reminds the owner of the service and is a happy and special talking point.

At the studio entrance door:

Presbyter: We come together for a holy and happy occasion. We have come to ask God's blessing on [*name*]'s new home.

(*Tracing the sign of the cross over the closed door*) In the name of the Holy Trinity: God our Father, Christ our Redeemer and the Holy Spirit the Comforter, Peace to this home.

People: Amen. God, we pray that the joy of your presence may enfold [*name*] here in [*his or her*] new home.

Presbyter: Blessed be God who gives peace and shelter.

(*The resident opens the door and moves into the new home.*)

Resident: Welcome to my new home. You are my family and friends. Your loving shows me God's loving.

Presbyter: [*Name*], The Lord watch over your going out and coming in.

All: **Amen.**

Resident: Please come in with me.

(*In the living room*)

Presbyter: Lord God, you have made us to need each other and to grow best with companions; bless this room and all those who shall eat or sit or talk or read or sing or pray here. May they share your care and understanding. In Jesus' name.

All: **Amen.**

Resident: Dear God, you never forget us. You will always be with me here in my new home, loving and caring for me as you have all my life long.

People: **We, your family and friends will not forget you either, [*name*]. It will be our joy to visit you here. We will pray for you and ask that you will pray for us.**

(*At the kitchen area*)

Presbyter: Lord, you provide for our daily bread. Bless this space and facilities for toast and tea making. May this place remind us that you are present in ordinary everyday things. Help us all to be people of genuine hospitality.

All: **Amen.**

(*At the bedroom space*)

Presbyter: (*Making the sign of the cross over the bed*)
              God of the darkness and the night, bless this sleeping place for [*name*]. Here may [*he or she*] know your loving presence, find rest for her tiredness and peace from all anxiety.
              Keep this place from all harm.

All: **Amen. May your holy angels guard [*name*] as [*he or she*] sleeps. O God, may your continual blessing strengthen [*him or her*]. Amen.**

(*If the Holy Communion is to be celebrated, the table may be set now. The service would follow the short liturgy given in Appendix 4. Otherwise the presbyter pronounces a suitable blessing, such as* 'The grace of the Lord Jesus Christ, the love of God and the fellowship of the Holy Spirit be with us all' (2 Corinthians 13:14) *or* 'May the God of hope fill you with all joy and peace in believing so that you may abound in hope by the power of the Holy Spirit' (Romans 15:13).

Appendix 8

A guide for pastors

Here is a check-list of ways by which the pastor (clergy, deacon or lay person) can take the initiative in pastoral visiting.

1. Wear something that may cue the person's remote memory of who you might be and of your role. Clergy should wear the clerical collar and lay pastors could wear a cross large enough to be seen by a person with impaired vision. A name badge will also be helpful.

2. Declare yourself at each visit (and never expect that people will remember you):

    -   I am…

    -   I come from…(a photograph or a picture of the church may help)

    -   I am visiting you

    -   I bring to you the love of our church family

    -   I would like to show you this…(church paper, bulletin, newsletter, anything with pictures. Look at these together. Take up responses. Make comments, one at a time).

3. Take with you something that may cue the person's remote memory. This could be a bunch of flowers from your garden, a music cassette (and player, of course), a photo album or book which illustrates aspects of life which may have been experienced decades ago.

4. Take the Bible and read a verse or two if this is appropriate. Choose carefully: verses should reinforce God's love and mercy rather than judgement. Be very intentional in your preparation. Identify, from your knowledge and understanding of the person, what it is you hope and pray will remain to comfort and strengthen them. It may be a verse that is very well known, for example, 'The Lord is my shepherd, I shall not want' (Psalm 23:1). I have found that many people are helped if I print a verse in large letters on card and leave it with them. Often I have returned to find the card propped up in a prominent

place and it is obvious that it is frequently read. I have also written blessings for people in the same way and these too are appreciated. Eventually, of course, depending on the area of brain loss, the ability to read is lost. Nevertheless this practice is very helpful for those whose cognitive abilities permit them to understand their prognosis.

5. Always pray with the person. I ask permission and have never been refused. A short, simple, direct, sentence prayer is appropriate as is the Lord's Prayer and, for Roman Catholics, the rosary. It is helpful to hold both hands of the elderly person while praying. This helps centre and 'hold' them in their attention to God and, of course, touching is good. A 'holding cross' is also helpful in aiding the person to centre in God.

6. Keep the visit short. Indicate you will be back and keep your promise. Go regularly, if possible at around the same time of the day and the same day of the week. Touch – embrace, kiss, shake hands, whatever is appropriate – as you leave.

7. Remember that although your visits are quickly forgotten, the good feelings remain with the person with Alzheimer's disease.

8. If possible keep in contact with the family or they may not know you visit. The confused person is not likely to remember to tell them. But your visits will encourage the care givers.

9. Be prepared to act as an advocate for the person with family, friends, care home or local authority departments. In this regard consult other professionals such as the social worker or Alzheimer's Society. Know the facts.

10. Pray for the person regularly. The pastor's work as intercessor is a primary pastoral work. Pray for the person's near kin and for yourself. Take special intercessions to the church family for corporate prayer.

11. The pastor and care giver will be helped by a proper understanding of the factors necessary for the nurture of spiritual well-being. This will include finding opportunities for the person with a dementia illness to sense, even momentarily, his or her own identity, experience relationship with others, self and the source of all being and to foster those activities which work towards the provision of a sense of meaning and purpose in one's life.

Visiting the person with dementia

This appendix offers a guide to visiting which is the new challenge for the family care giver. This may be used by clergy and others as the basis for teaching the care giver new skills in order to maintain relationship with the dementing person for as long as possible. The original is in pamphlet format (obtainable from MHA Care Group, Epworth House, Stuart Street, Derby DE1 2EQ) and may be copied with acknowledgement to the author.

Some suggestions for those who care
Understanding dementia
Dementia is caused by a physical change in brain structure.

Dementia types

- Alzheimer's disease
- alcohol-related dementia
- multi-infarct dementia – a series of small strokes.

Dementia causes a decline in a person's ability to

- remember
- think
- reason.

People with dementia
are unable to cope with the usual visiting mode.

The visitor
needs to take the initiative for successful communication.

Communicating
with others is a basic human need.

Visiting

the person with dementia is a challenge to communicate in ways appropriate to the person's diminishing abilities.

Visiting

is for nourishing love and relationships.

Useful visiting tools are

- orientation: name, time, season, place and weather
- memory cueing: smell, music, colour, pictures, texture, and so on
- feelings: people with dementia continue to respond to feelings long after they are no longer able to understand
- 'the shortest distance between two people is a smile'
- declaring yourself: 'I am Joan. I am your wife. I have come to visit you, Bob. You are my husband. I love you. We are at Sunnyview Hospital. You live here. I am visiting you.'
- using simple sentences
- speaking slowly and clearly
- waiting for a response – the person with dementia needs time to frame an answer
- avoiding questions
- using self-included humour
- learning not to fear silence
- using non-verbal modes of communication – touch, gesture
- trying to maintain eye contact
- walking with the person or the wheelchair
- saying if you do not understand the person – ask for the statement to be repeated and if this triggers upset use your best guess (guesswork at least means the dementia person is being taken seriously)
- assuming that there is capacity for insight
- taking something which may memory cue the person – a photograph, a tape of a once-favourite song, something the person once made, and so on
- keeping your visit short

- visiting regularly, if possible same day of week and same time – constancy promotes orientation
- indicating you will be back and keeping your promise.

After visiting

Try to identify any strong feelings in yourself. Then:

- acknowledge
- share
- plan.

Action helps 'ground' feelings

Positive follow-ups to help nourish your own total well-being include:

- gardening
- walking
- talking it over.

References

Adler. A. (1921) *The Neurotic Constitution.* London: Kegan Paul.

Adler, A. (1924) *The Practice and Theory of Individualistic Psychology and Psychotherapy.* London: Kegan Paul.

Bell, J. and McGregor, I. (1991) 'Living for the moment.' *Nursing Times 87,* 18.

Benland, C. (1988) 'The S-factor: Taha Wairua – the dimension of the human spirit.' In *Report of the Royal Commission on Social Policy,* New Zealand: Government Printer.

Blackhouse, H. (1985) (Author unknown) *The Cloud of Unknowing.* London: Hodder and Stoughton.

Board of Social Responsibility Report (1990) *Ageing.* London: Church House Publishing.

Brown, M. and Ellor, J.W. (1981) 'An approach to treatment of the symptoms caused by cognitive disorders in the aged.' *Salud Publica* 23.

Browning, R. (1912) 'Rabbi Ben Ezra.' In A. Wuiller-Couch *The Oxford Book of Victorian Verse.* Oxford: Oxford University Press, 1912.

Camus, A. (1955) *The Myth of Sisyphus.* New York: Vintage.

Cowley, J. (1989) *Aoteroa Psalms.* New Zealand: Catholic Supplies Ltd.

Davis, R. (1989) *My Journey into Alzheimer's Disease.* Wheaton Il: Tyndale.

de Mello, A. (1989) *The Heart of the Enlightened.* London: Collins Fount.

Erikson, E. (1963) *Childhood and Society.* New York: Norton.

Feil, N. (1993) *The Validation Breakthrough.* USA: Public Health Profession Press Inc.

Fish, S. (1990) *Alzheimer's Disease: Caring for your Loved Ones.* London: Lion.

'Food for thought – on caring' (1985) *World Federation of Occupational Therapists Bulletin 12.* November.

Frank, A. (1960) *The Diary of Anne Frank.* London: Hutchinson Educational.

Frankl, V. (1963) *Man's Search for Meaning.* Washington Square Press. Also (1964) London: Hodder and Stoughton.

Frankl, V. (1978) *Psychotherapy and Existentialism.* New York: Vintage Books. Also (1970) London: Souvenir Press.

Froggatt, A. and Shamy, E. (1994) *Dementia: A Christian Perspective.* Derby Christian Council on Ageing.

Guffey, R.W. Jr (1991) 'Oh to be so poor.' In *Alive Now,* May/June 1991.

Hanson, B.G. (1989) In *Family Process 28.*

Harrison, A. (ed) (1993) *Spiritual Needs of People with Dementia.* Stirling: DSDC

Illich, I. (1976) *Medical Nemesis: the expropriation of health.* London: Calder and Boyars.

Inimaera, W. (1986) *The Matriarch.* Auckland NZ: Heinemann.

James, W. (1950) *The Principles of Psychology* (pp.291–400). New York: Dover.

Julian of Norwich (1978) *Showings.* New York: Paulist Press.

Kimble, M.A. (1990) *Ageing and the Search for Meaning.* New York: Haworth Press.

Kitwood, T. and Bredin, K. (1992) *Person to Person, A Guide to the Care of Those with Failing Mental Powers.* Essex: Gale Centre.

Koopman-Boyden (ed) (1993) *New Zealand's Ageing Society, The Implications.* Wellington NZ: Daphne Brassell Associates Press.

Kushner, H. (1988) *When bad things happen to good people.* In J. Rupp, *Praying our Goodbyes,* Indiana: Ave Maria Press.

McClusky, H. (1981) In S.M. Grabowski (ed) *Preparing Educators of Adults.* San Francisco: Jossey-Bass.

Mandlen, E. (1985) *Will you take me home?* ADRA Newsletter.

Maslow, A. (1954) *Motivation and Personality.* New York: Harper and Row.

Milne, A.A. (1927) *Now We Are Six.* London: Methuen.

Nouwen, H.J.M. (1974) *Out of Solitatude – Three Meditations on the Christian Life.* Indiana: Ave Maria Press.

Nouwen, H.J.M. (1998) *The Living Reminder – Service and Prayer in Memory of Jesus Christ.* San Francisco: Harper and Row.

Opie, A. (ed) (1991) *Caring Alone: Looking after the Elderly Confused at Home.* Wellington NZ: Daphne Brassell Associates.

Paul, S.S. and Paul, J.A. (1994) *Humanity Comes of Age – The New Context of Ministry to the Elderly.* Geneva: World Council of Churches.

Peterson, E. (1993) *The Message.* Colorado Springs: Navpress.

Peterson, E. (1989) *The Contemplative Pastor – Returning to the Art of Spiritual Direction.* Grand Rapids Michigan: Erdmans.

Petzsch, H. (1984) *Does He Know How Frightening He is in His Strangeness? A Study in Attitudes to Dementing People.* Edinburgh: Department of Ethics and Practical Theology.

Potok, C. (1990) *Davita's Harp.* Maryland USA: Fawcett Colombine.

Potok, C. (1972) *My Name is Asher Lev.* New York: Alfred A Knopf. London: Penguin.

Pratt, C., Schmall, V. and Wright, S.D. (1985) 'Spiritual support for care-givers of dementing patients.' In *Journal of Religion and Health 24,* 1.

Riesberg, B. (1983) *Alzheimer's Disease: The Standard Reference.* New York: Free Press.

Stokes, G. and Goudie, F. (1990) *Working with Dementia.* Bicester: Winslow.

Vanstone, W. (1982) *The Stature of Waiting.* London: DLT.

Wilson, H.S. (1989) 'Family care-giving for a relative with Alzheimer's dementia: coping with negative choices.' *Nursing Research Journal 38,* 2.

All scripture quotations unless otherwise acknowledged are from the New Revised Standard Version of the Bible (Reference Edition), copyright 1989 by the Division of Christian Education of the National Council of the Churches of Christ in the USA.